THE MAN WHO SAVED THE WORLD FROM SMALLPOX

THE MAN WHO SAVED THE WORLD FROM SMALLPOX

◆

DOCTOR EDWARD JENNER

A Novel

GEORGE F. SMITH, M.D.

iUniverse, Inc.
New York Lincoln Shanghai

THE MAN WHO SAVED THE WORLD FROM SMALLPOX
DOCTOR EDWARD JENNER

All Rights Reserved © 2004 by George F Smith

No part of this book may be reproduced or transmitted in any form or by any means, graphic, electronic, or mechanical, including photocopying, recording, taping, or by any information storage retrieval system, without the written permission of the publisher.

iUniverse, Inc.

For information address:
iUniverse, Inc.
2021 Pine Lake Road, Suite 100
Lincoln, NE 68512
www.iuniverse.com

ISBN: 0-595-32957-8

Printed in the United States of America

DEDICATION: TO MY BELOVED EDITOR

Patricia N. Smith

Contents

PROLOGUE 1
CHAPTER 1 3
CHAPTER 2 6
CHAPTER 3 14
CHAPTER 4 21
CHAPTER 5 34
CHAPTER 6 46
CHAPTER 7 53
CHAPTER 8 62
CHAPTER 9 69
CHAPTER 10 80
CHAPTER 11 94
CHAPTER 12 106
CHAPTER 13 115
CHAPTER 14 127
CHAPTER 15 136
CHAPTER 16 146
CHAPTER 17 155
CHAPTER 18 163

CHAPTER 19 172
CHAPTER 20 183
CHAPTER 21 197
CHAPTER 22 207
CHAPTER 23 221
CHAPTER 24 239
EPILOGUE 251

PROLOGUE

❖

The beautiful Nana dies of Smallpox

She was fruit of the charnel-house, a heap of matter and blood, a shovelful of corrupted flesh thrown down on the pillow. The pustules had invaded the whole of the face, so that each touched its neighbour. Fading and sunken, they had assumed the greyish hue of mud, and on that formless pulp, where the features had ceased to be traceable, they already resembled some decaying damp from the grave. One eye, the left eye, had completely foundered among bubbling purulence, and the other, which remained half open, looked like a deep black ruinous hole. The nose was still suppurating. Quite a reddish crust was peeling from one of the cheeks, and invading the mouth, which it distorted into a horrible grin. And over this loathsome and grotesque mask of death, the hair, the beautiful hair, still blazed like sunlight and flowed downwards in the rippling gold. Venus was rotting. It looked as if the poison she had assimilated in the gutters, left there by the roadside, the ferment with which she had poisoned a whole people, had now reached to her face and turned it to corruption.

Nana
By Emile Zola 1840–1902

1

THERE ARE, MOST ASSUREDLY, multiple reasons for writing a story, and undoubtedly stories, such as those of the bible, were ignited by the prerequisite of spiritual passion; other stories may be written out of anger, bitterness or, of course, vanity or cupidity. Besides, writing about another person, or some entity, invariably renders meaning to oneself. Also, there appears to be a congenital need in many to put their thoughts on paper, for whatever reason. For my part, the emotion for writing this story was guilt.

Having lived in England—to be more exact, London—for a number of years, and having spent many hours in the numerous, excellent medical and scientific libraries available, I could not help but become familiar with an eighteenth century doctor who *saved the world* from the dread disease, *smallpox*. This malady, which yearly destroyed a large part of the world's population left many, who did not die from its ravages, disfigured by facial scarring and pitting, while others were condemned to be forever blind. While the *plague* was a greater killer when it struck, it killed quickly, and if an individual was fortunate enough to survive, there were no deforming lesions or stigmas.

Whereas much has been written about smallpox vaccination, less emphasis has been placed upon the man, Doctor Edward Jenner, who discovered and promoted its use. To fully appreciate the devastating and chilling effect that smallpox had on the world's population, it is necessary to examine what happened before and after Jenner's remarkable discovery.

To be sure, great discoveries are inevitably associated with great hardships. This is the story of a man, a very special type of man, who refused to be diverted from finding a way to save the world from a horrible disease, smallpox. It was a pestilence, a profanation against the whole of the human race, and he wished to subjugate it and obliterate it from this earth. He demonstrated how smallpox could be prevented, and he speculated that the disease could be eliminated from this earth, if it were deprived of its only source of nourishment—human beings.

On his voyage of discovery, Doctor Jenner worked alone, using his own financial resources and whatever little time he could purloin from his busy country practice of medicine. How different it is today for research workers, sheltered in huge modern laboratories, surrounded by obliging laboratory assistants, and most essential of all, smothered by bountiful mountains of governmental funds.

Over the years, my sense of guilt remained because there was not enough written about Doctor Jenner the man, although much was published about the disease, smallpox, that he had tamed. Once I became familiar with the man, it was obvious that there was something unimaginable about his supreme sacrifice, and that by accomplishing the inconceivable, he had set an example for future generations of doctors and healers to emulate.

While this story is about a real individual, still, it is not a biography. Biographies, in general, are written by trained historians who follow exacting rules and customs. This story was never meant to be a biography, but merely a novel, a story about a doctor who was a product of his environment, the eighteenth century—a very special century.

It is challenging today to write about someone who lived over two centuries ago, since we live at a time when the world seems to be spinning at a frenetic pace, and history, to many, is nothing more than something that happened only yesterday. To compensate for this deficiency, the writer has elected to present Jenner's place in history in the form of a simple story, in the hope that it would be more acceptable to the reader.

It is difficult—nay, impossible—for our society to believe, as Isaac Newton once said, when questioned about his remarkable discoveries, "I can see so far because I am standing on the shoulders of giants." Of course his giants included Galileo and all the wonderful mathematicians who preceded him. Jenner, too, had his own giants and, in the process of furthering medical science, he became a giant to others who followed. But Jenner's story is not just the story of smallpox and vaccination; it is the story of the human race and the interdependence that we have on one another, since vaccination saved everyone regardless of race, skin color or the continent upon which a person lived. Jenner's discovery could have occurred anywhere in the world. It just happened, at that time in the history of scientific discoveries, that Jenner was an Englishman. At another time, in the long evolution of man, the discovery could have occurred in a different country or on another continent. History is not events; it is people, and perhaps Jenner's real contribution was not just the discovery of vaccination, but the example that he set by freely sharing his discovery and his knowledge with all who asked, regardless who they were or where they lived.

The reader must know that the only real people in this story are Jenner and the people of his generation. The modern-day individuals attempting to tell the story are fictitious—figments of the imagination.

The author has taken certain liberties. For example, whenever possible, Doctor Jenner's spoken words are taken from his copious letters, but at times, his words are paraphrased; and for the sake of comprehension or continuity of the plot, the dialogue consists of what the author speculated could have been said. Be advised, however, that this suppositional device and rearrangement of events, for better continuity of the story, are luxuries peculiar to the storyteller but denied to the true historian.

My story starts with the death of an innocent seaman on board a Spanish ship, heading for Cuba, but the real story took place at a dinner party, at a marvelous sixteenth century English country home. So let us begin.

2

THE YEAR: 1518; THE SHIP: THE SANTA ROSA; the Port: Cadiz, Spain. Christopher Columbus sailed from the Port of Palos, in 1492, on his search for a westerly route to the Orient, and the Santa Rosa followed that same route to the Canary Islands, nearly thirty years later.

It really wasn't a New World that was discovered but, at that time, the people of Europe spoke as if there were an Old World and a New World. In truth, the worlds were the same age. Nevertheless, there was a quantum difference between them. The Old World had been exploited and exfoliated, during the millennia it had been inhabited, while the New World was pristine and protected by its inhabitants; the Old World was filled with putrefaction and corruption, and the New World was free of Old World germs and human waste; the Old World was full of decadence and disease, and the New World was free of degeneracy and degradation; the Old World was raped of its trees, and the New World had an abundance of forests with trees that were worshipped as if they were gods; the Old World was built upon prejudice and thralldom—a group of countries which confused technical advancements with human and spiritual perfection; in the New World, spirituality bound the tribes together to form nations. From then on the Old World would empty its pollution, its germs, onto a primitive New World, in which sin was lacking and repentance wasn't needed.

The port at Palos, Spain was a well known harbor that supplied merchant ships and sailors who carried on the rich commerce of Spain. Of course, its great fame was that it supplied the men and ships for Columbus' voyage of discovery and conquest.

The ship, the Santa Rosa, a Spanish galleon was a large sailing vessel that could be used as either a warship or a merchantman, depending on its fittings and rigging. For her time, she was considered an imposing sailing ship, with three or four masts and a high forecastle and stern. In the stern were the Captain's cabin and work area, and a closet-size room for the physician, plus a slightly larger cabin nearby shared by the three officers. The crew lived, slept and cooked underneath the high deck of the forecastle which was only partially enclosed. The open section exposed the crew to the elements: rain, snow, heat and cold. Thirty passengers shared a small dormitory-like area below the main deck, in the stern of the ship. It was there, with little or no privacy, that they slept, cooked, ate, eliminated their bodily waste, and made love. There was a crew of thirty seamen, three officers, the physician and the Captain. The Santa Rosa's trip to Cuba, would take two to two-and-a-half months depending upon the currents and the winds. Her cargo consisted of agricultural products from Malaga; leather from Cordova; iron products such as pots, pan, plates, and battle armor, including swords from Toledo; and tools for farming and irrigation. The vessel was to be loaded, on its return voyage, with tobacco and coca, products that were eagerly sought after by the Europeans.

On the morning the ship set sail from Cadiz, an ominous sign was seen as they left the harbor. A brief thunder and lightning storm passed over the city, and as it did, a bolt of lightning struck the steeple of the Sailors' Church setting it on fire. The crew interpreted the lightning strike as a warning sign, but they were uncertain what it signified. Some suggested that since the lightning struck the church where the sailors received a blessing on the morning before they sailed, it could be an omen that disease—perhaps plague or smallpox—had entered the city and was aboard the vessel. The Captain ignored the crew's remarks; he wasn't a superstitious man. Besides, if it were a sign that smallpox was present, he wasn't worried, because most of the crew had had the disease and survived. The skin on their faces revealed the scars and pockmarks, indications that they had had smallpox and were now immune. For the passengers, it was a different story. There were fourteen adults, a few showing evidence of having had the disease, and sixteen children, ranging from three days to twelve years of age, none of whom had ever been exposed to smallpox.

The sea was calm and the weather was balmy, as the ship left the port and sailed south, but all was not well on board the ship, as she headed for the New World. The superstitious crewmen felt it in their guts. They knew that there was trouble ahead, but they didn't know what to expect. The officers, and even the Captain, felt uneasy about the voyage, but he unceremoniously passed it off by telling himself that all crews, at the start of a long and dangerous journey, had premonitions about not returning.

For the first week, many of the adult passengers were deadly seasick, but the children fared well on the trip. Both the passengers and crew rejoiced when they saw land on the horizon for the first time. It was the Canary Islands, the only stop before sailing westward, as so many ships before them had done, on their way to the New World.

Since the ship was badly in need of repairs and some additional sails, it would remain in port for a week, during which time the passengers and crew were free to explore the town and the hills. Provisions, such as, water, food, and wine stocks would be replenished while the repairs were being made.

The passengers especially the children, enjoyed exploring the town and running in the hills. But for the crew, whose needs were different, their time was spent in the taverns, drinking and seeking out the fun-loving women who welcomed their company. Unbeknownst to the sailors, some of their playmates recently had been exposed to smallpox by sailors from another ship anchored in the harbor.

After seven days in the Canary Islands, the ship again put out to sea. This time, she steered boldly to the tip of the Canary Islands, where she would trap in her sails the westerly winds that would take her to Cuba. The ship was soon in uncharted seas, and many of the uninitiated members of the crew, who sailed these waters for the first time, were uncertain and apprehensive. There were times when the crew wanted to turn back and even thought of mutiny, but the Captain dauntlessly held his course.

And so, the difficult and dangerous part of the voyage began. The Spanish galleon, the Santa Rosa, was similar to many such ships in the Spanish Armada that, later in the century, would recklessly attempt to conquer England. The Armada failed. It was a poorly conceived plan that would badly weaken the Spanish and their dream of world dominance; and start the English navy on a shipbuilding program that would enable her to rule the seas for the next five centuries.

The westerly winds were brisk and the current was favorable, as the ship sailed quietly through the waters of the South Atlantic Ocean. But time would prove that the crew's fears were justified; there was trouble lying in wait for them. Within the hull was an invisible threat, a virus that would soon infect the ship's crew and passengers and, eventually, conquer and destroy a large part of the indigenous populations of the New World.

The ship's doctor, a Spanish nobleman, dressed meticulously in a uniform of the rank of captain, was accompanied by his servant as he responded to a call to see a sick crew member. By now, it was nearly three weeks since the ship had left the Canary Islands, and four days before, the seaman had developed a fever, muscle aches and pains, and was too weak to perform his duties. He was allowed to remain on his bed of straw. It was thought that he would soon recover, but his condition deteriorated and the doctor was summoned.

By the time the doctor and his servant saw the patient, he was beyond help. He was sweating profusely, in a semi-conscious state and moaning with pain. His skin was a bright reddish hue, and there were telltale small, pearly pustules covering the exposed parts of his body, mainly his face and hands. On closer examination, there were similar lesions covering his eyes and the lining of his mouth and throat.

The cause of the man's distress was immediately obvious. The pustules were those of the dreaded smallpox, and he, obviously, had a severe form of the disease. There was no cure; the man was doomed, and in a matter of days, he would be dead. They both knew this, but only the doctor had any idea of the devastation that was about to be caused aboard the ship. While the physician could do nothing to save the man, he wanted to try to make the poor soul comfortable. He directed his servant to sponge the man to control his fever, and offer him sips of water to moisten his parched lips and throat. Neither the doctor nor his servant had concerns for themselves, since both had had the disease and were immune.

The most important thing that the doctor ordered his servant to do was to isolate the man in a quiet area of the ship, and to hang a canvas curtain so that the man could not be seen by the crew or the passengers. The servant was then ordered to remain with the seaman until he died.

Returning to his cabin, the physician sat at his desk, overwhelmed with powerlessness. He was troubled, not merely over the impending death of one unknown seaman, but because he knew what a terrible contagious disease was incubating in him and, undoubtedly, in other members of the crew and passengers. Once the seaman died, the putrefaction and pestilence would reappear on board the ship. The doctor was also concerned that the disease would be brought into Cuba and result in a catastrophic epidemic. His thoughts were now for the well-being of the Indians of Cuba, the island for which the ship was heading. He shuddered to think what could happen to this unprotected population of innocent Indians, once they came into contact with smallpox.

The doctor ordered that after the seaman died, his diseased remains be secretly dumped overboard, sans the prayers of his fellow seamen. Every precaution was to be taken so as not to alarm the crew or the passengers. The servant alone was to enclose the body in a canvas sack and cast it, at night, into the sea. The physician had hoped to dispose of the body before the pustules could be observed by anyone aboard the ship, including the Captain. His plan was to say the man died of chickenpox, notwithstanding if there were similar deaths on board the ship, the hoax couldn't be sustained.

It wasn't long, however, before one after another, half the adults and all the children on board the ship developed smallpox. The crew was more fortunate, since only three seamen were affected. The rest had had smallpox and were now immune. Before the ship arrived in Cuba, of those who had contracted the disease, one-third of the adults and all of the children had died. The three crewmen who were afflicted all survived.

Based upon his medical experience and common sense, the doctor insisted that, when the ship dropped anchor in Santiago de Cuba Harbor, no one be allowed to disembark, until there were no new cases of smallpox for at least two weeks. The ship's Captain, however, wouldn't listen to such nonsense; hadn't the crew and passengers suffered enough during this long and laborious voyage, without having them detained while the ship remained at anchor in the harbor? Perhaps the Captain also had monetary reasons for wanting to move on; the ship was scheduled to both unload and take on precious cargo at other Cuban ports. Failure to maintain scheduled appointments meant a financial loss for both the ship's owners and the Captain. And once again, in man's journey on earth, power and authority superseded common sense and knowledge; the surviving passengers and some of the crew disembarked without delay in Santiago de Cuba. The ship then proceeded to move on to Havana and other ports. Havana, at that time, was slightly larger than a fishing village, but the ship was able to take on fresh water and salted fish as provisions, as well as buy tobacco and coca to sell back in Spain.

As the doctor predicted, some of the disembarking passengers and crew were carrying the deadly smallpox virus in their throats, and even though they were not sick at the time, they were incubating the disease. Shortly after the Santa Rosa sailed, a convoy of other ships was getting ready to leave for the coast of what was then named New Spain. Some of the Santa Rosa's crew members signed on as seamen on one of the ships headed by the expedition's leader, Hernando Cortes. When Cortes was ready to leave on his journey of conquest, several of the former Santa Rosa seamen, unknowingly, infected some of Cortes' crew with smallpox.

Cortes provisioned his ships with fresh water, cassava bread, wine and salt fish and pork. The only live animals that were loaded were war horses, and swine for food. These were the only domesticated animals in Cuba, at that time. In addition, Cortes had the ships well stocked with protective armor, guns, powder, crossbows, pikes, spikes, lances and other munitions, all items to be used for war and conquest, rather than for friendly trade.

Hernando Cortes was born a gentleman, having descended from titled ancestors, on both sides of his family. He took great pains with the preparation of his fleet, but was forced to hurry things along for fear that his father-in-law, the governor, Diego Velazquez, would prevent him from sailing. Malice and envy reigned among the Velazquez relatives, who were offended because their kinsman-by-marriage, Cortes, neither trusted nor listened to them.

Early in February, 1519, Cortes had his crews of Spanish conquistadors secretly taken aboard their ships, at night; and shortly thereafter, they sailed out of the port of Santiago de Cuba on his crusade of conquest.

The die was cast. The New World was to be infected by one of the most deadly diseases known to the Old World, smallpox. The course was charted as if on a nautical map. The Santa Rosa left Palos, Spain, and stopped at the Canary Islands to pick up fresh provisions. An unwanted "stowaway," smallpox, which had been dropped off at Santiago de Cuba, boarded one of Cortes' ships for a quick and easy ride to the port of Vera Cruz, in the New World. There it made its way ashore and permanently altered the history of mankind.

And from that time onward, the Indians in the New World would die by the millions, and many of its cherished tribes would vanish from the face of the earth. With the aid of an infinitesimal smallpox virus, the Old World would be able to conquer and control two continents of the New World with relative ease.

3

ON A NIPPY JANUARY EVENING, Professor Lawrence Penfield, a dedicated biologist and mathematician, was enjoying an evening dinner with his wife, Iris, and three colleagues and their wives, at his large 16th century country home. Actually, the majestic Tudor home no longer belonged to the professor, since he had given it to The National Trust of England as a national treasure, but he still had the use of it during his lifetime. He enjoyed using the house on weekends, seeing that it permitted him the luxury of leaving the noisy, polluted confines of London, and taking long, leisurely walks in the countryside with his family and weekend guests.

A few of the children of the guests also were invited for the weekend. Professor Penfield thoughtfully arranged for a neighbor, who was a teacher, to entertain them, both indoors and outdoors, while their parents were with the Prof and his wife. But Prof also enjoyed spending some time with the children, because, as he said, he liked to "watch the wheels going round in their heads." On those occasions, one could see his delight in being stumped, if only momentarily, by some of their questions.

The children relished their weekend at Prof's house and, of course, Prof made sure it was a rewarding, educational experience for them.

As was their custom, the Penfields and their guests dined in a spacious and stately country-style kitchen. The large, wooden, rectangular table and chairs were made of the finest oak. The chairs were ponderous and cumbersome; nevertheless, they were comfortable. A middle-aged married couple, who were caretakers when the Penfields were in London, prepared and served the meal. The man and wife had been in the service of the Penfields for the past twenty years and resided at the beautiful, old house, full-time, year-in and year-out. They enjoyed working for the Prof and his wife, but they didn't appear to be very happy catering to the guests.

The cuisine was good, old-country-style English cooking. Naturally, Sherry wine was served, and there were casual conversations occurring before sitting down to the meal. The purpose of the Sherry wine, of course, was to relax everyone and to prepare both their minds and their stomachs for the good things they were about to receive. But most satisfying of all, the ceremony was simple and relaxing.

Bowls and platters of food were placed on the table and the guests were expected to pass them to each other and serve themselves. At the same time, the professor placed two decanters of wine, one white and one red, on the table for all to enjoy with their meal. While the food may have been less than memorable, the conversation and the ambience were always engaging and thought-provoking. As was his way of doing things, the professor beckoned the group to begin the meal with a toast. Still, it seemed inappropriate to hail the Queen yet once again, for the hundredth time, so he suggested that they toast Doctor Edward Jenner who had died on this same date, January 24th, one hundred and eighty years earlier, in the year 1823.

Could it be that the professor was so agile with dates because he was a mathematician and liked numbers? The explanation is simpler than that. Prof knew that date, since it was his hobby to delve into medical history, and Doctor Edward Jenner was one of his preferred individuals and an ideal subject of conversation.

First and foremost, the professor carefully reminded the diners that without Jenner's discovery of smallpox vaccination, three or four people present at the meal that evening wouldn't be alive to be wined, dined and partake in the conversation. This remark didn't go unattended by those who understood its meaning, so the standard "Hear, hear!" was their immediate response.

After the meal, the group moved into a cavernous living room with a huge open fireplace at one end of the room, its blazing logs beckoning the guests to draw near. The women, in particular, relished being close to the hearth with its radiating heat, considering that they were less warmly dressed than the men. Away from the fire, the room was chilly and somewhat uncomfortable, inasmuch as the house was unheated.

The professor explained to his guests, as he had done numerous times before, that he was unable to add central heat to the house, because of the fragile condition of the building with its the old, dried-out beams supporting the structure. The group knew the explanation for the cold rooms, and accepted the rustic living conditions, as part of a consequence of spending an otherwise pleasurable weekend with the professor and his charming wife.

At this point, the caretaker appeared with a large decanter of vintage Port wine. He filled eight small glasses, which he then served to the Penfields and their six guests. The liquid was a double-barreled delight; it sweetened the palate and, at the same time, appeared to warm the body as it was assimilated into the blood stream.

The guests seated themselves on two long sofas that faced each other and were separated by a large coffee table. Iris, the professor's wife, sat in an over-stuffed chair close to the fireplace, while the professor stood alongside the hearth, with one arm resting on the mantel. Thus the discussion began with the professor, as usual, selecting the topic of conversation.

The Prof personified the typical English "absent-minded professor." However, this professor forgot only those things that he considered of little value or that he totally disagreed with; everything else was locked into his brain, as if carved in granite. He was in his mid-sixties; slightly shorter than most men—perhaps five feet five inches tall; on the soft side, without being pudgy. His strength and distinction resided in the upper one-sixth of his body: his head and neck. His extremely pleasant face, without distinguishing marks, was what everyone focused upon, considering that most of the time his facial expressions were amiable and engaging. He had a substantial skull covered with thin, wavy, dark hair, its wide streaks of grey only adding to his unconventional overall appearance. No one was ever quite sure who his haberdasher was, or if he even had one; and he certainly didn't buy his suits and shoes at the leading men's shops in central London, even though he could well afford it. Only when he was giving or attending a lecture, did he wear a respectable black suit; otherwise, his wardrobe was restricted to a thick, slightly frayed tweed jacket, plain white shirt and a poorly knotted tie that was usually askew. His trousers seemed baggy, some shade between gray and black, held up by a belt fastened haphazardly outside of and below the belt-loops. He was the perfect, brilliant but absent-minded professor, who beguiled all who crossed his path.

The professor had had a distinguished career in both biology and mathematics, and came from a brilliant family that was both wealthy and talented. He was educated at Eaton and went on to Christ Church College, Oxford, where he took honors in both biology and mathematics and, eventually, obtained a doctor's degree in medicine. Later, he did advanced work in mathematics in Germany, before returning to University College London, where he was appointed Professor of Biology. His publications and books were legend, and he was ultimately honored by being elected to the Royal Society, England's most prestigious institution.

"Perhaps," said the Prof, "since Doctor Jenner's name was mentioned at the dinner table, we could carry on by discussing his career. He was an exceptional person, you know, and a controversial one at that. But anyone who has ever accomplished anything of consequence is, *ipso facto*, controversial."

Professor Foxworth, who was in the Prof's department, and a man of authority himself, interjected, "While Jenner had his detractors or, more precisely, critics and enemies in England, he was always a hero and a savior in Europe and most other countries throughout the world. Maybe, Prof, you can explain to us why the doctors in England had such difficulty accepting Jenner's discovery, while doctors and scientists in other countries venerated him for his demonstration that vaccination, using the serum extract of cowpox, prevented a person from developing the smallpox disease."

As was his custom, Professor Penfield was slow to answer the question, and spent an indeterminate amount of time meditating, before starting the conversation again. "Well...there is no simple answer, Cedric," meaning Professor Foxworth. "Anyone who proposes a totally original idea or makes a new discovery isn't necessarily a hero in his time. History is replete with individuals who made major contributions to our pool of knowledge, only to be scorned during their lifetime but honored for them after they died. Take, for instance, Gregory Mendel and his discovery of genetics. His ideas were so complex and original that his fellow scientists had no concept what he was talking about; consequently, the poor man died thinking that he was a complete failure. As a contemporary example, Cedric, if someone requested money for a research project that was so new and original that there was nothing with which to compare it, our governmental bureaucrats would, most likely, not support the project. In general, it is hard on an individual who is far ahead of the scientific thinking of the time. Remember the grief and animosity that Pasteur and Galileo were subjected to, for proposing new ideas. Pasteur was castigated by the doctors, and Galileo was imprisoned in his home by the Vatican authorities. No Cedric, you can't get too far ahead of the contemporary scientific thinking, without expecting to be subjected to some abuse. For Jenner's detractors, there were other factors also operating, namely, jealousy and even greed, but we will get to that later.

"Fortunately, Cedric, cases of smallpox are, theoretically, nonexistent today. I am sure that none of us has ever seen a patient with severe manifestations of the disease."

The Professor then walked across the room to a walled bookcase and removed a small book entitled "Nana," by Emile Zola. He returned to his place by the fire and addressed the group, "Zola, who was born in 1840, less than two decades after Jenner died, wrote a vivid and dismal portrayal of severe smallpox. Let me read it to you, so that you will be able to understand what we are talking about this evening."

With that, he began to read, "The beautiful Nana dies of Smallpox. She was fruit of the charnel-house, a heap of matter and blood, a shovelful of corrupted flesh thrown down on the pillow. The pustules had invaded the whole of the face, so that each touched its neighbour. Fading and sunken, they had assumed the greyish hue of mud, and on that formless pulp, where the features had ceased to be traceable, they already resembled some decaying damp from the grave. One eye, the left eye, had completely foundered among bubbling purulence, and the other, which remained half open, looked like a deep black ruinous hole. The nose was still suppurating. Quite a reddish crust was peeling from one of the cheeks, and invading the mouth, which it distorted into a horrible grin. And over this loathsome and grotesque mask of death, the hair, the beautiful hair, still blazed like sunlight and flowed downwards in the rippling gold. Venus was rotting. It looked as if the poison she had assimilated in the gutters, left there by the roadside, the ferment with which she had poisoned a whole people, had now reached to her face and turned it to corruption."

Prof closed the book and laid it on the mantel. He turned to the group and said, "Zola's story gives us a clear picture of what humanity was faced with, before Jenner came on the scene. Now, let us discuss what was known about smallpox in those trying times.

"By the start…"

◆ ◆ ◆

By the start of the seventeenth century, smallpox was widespread throughout England and, for that matter, Europe and Asia; even the New World wasn't spared. The disease was imported into the Caribbean by Columbus' sailors in 1492, and it eventually was spread from Cuba to Mexico by the soldiers and crew of the conquistador, Hernando Cortes, in 1519. By the beginning of the eighteenth century, smallpox was well represented in North, South and Central Americas. Without a doubt, the disease spread easily in the Americas, where the indigenous populations had no natural immunity against it.

Many of the men with Columbus and Cortes had had smallpox before they sailed. In their responses to being exposed to smallpox, there were major differences between the sailors and the Indians in the New World. The conquistadors who had smallpox, during childhood, and survived it, were left with immunity to protect them against the disease; but the Indian populations of the Americas, having never been exposed to the disease, had no immunity to protect them. When the conquistadors brought smallpox to these isolated populations, the death rates were extremely high; in some tribes the entire population died of the disease.

When smallpox first entered Europe, about the thirteenth century, the death rate was appalling, but over the centuries, as people survived the disease and developed immunity to it, the death rate dropped to a steady 30 percent of all those who were infected, and by then, most of the deaths were in young children.

Smallpox in England, even during Jenner's time, spread quickly throughout the cities and villages and continued to be a dreadful killer. The disease was more feared than the plague, which efficiently and effectively destroyed its victim in three to four days. Those who succumbed to smallpox suffered a slow death—taking, perhaps, two weeks or more. And the death wasn't merciful; the patient's body slowly rotted away, particularly the facial area. Moreover, if the victim survived, the face could be scarred and disfigured by the pitted depressions that remained after the dried crusts fell off. For a woman, it was a horrible experience. Her beauty would have disappeared forever. Blindness or marked visual impairment often followed the illness. In England, during the eighteenth century, there were towns and villages in which nearly the entire populations had facial scarring or pitting, as the result of having had smallpox.

4

STANDING BEFORE THE FIREPLACE, the Professor seemed lost in his thoughts. His guests waited patiently for him to decide which part of Jenner's life they would discuss. Prof sensed that they were starting to get fidgety, and he said, "It has occurred to me that, before getting too far along, we should follow Socrates' advice and define some of the words that we shall be using this evening. It's important, if we are to understand one another.

"In the early part of the eighteenth century, before Jenner, the only protection against naturally occurring smallpox was achieved by inoculating a small amount of smallpox matter into the skin. The smallpox matter contained viral particles in a weakened state so that, hopefully, the recipient would develop a mild form of the disease, without becoming seriously ill. This method of producing immunity was termed *smallpox inoculation*. Since this was the only procedure of this type, until 1798, it was referred to simply as *inoculation*. Sometime later, smallpox inoculation was also referred to as *variolation*. Therefore, this evening, these two terms—inoculation and variolation—will be used interchangeably.

"In 1798, Jenner published the results of his discovery that the inoculation of cowpox into the skin produced immunity against the disease, smallpox. In the publication, he referred to this practice as cowpox inoculation. But, because of the similarity in the terms, smallpox inoculation and cowpox inoculation, the latter was referred to simply as vaccination. The word, vaccine, was derived from the Latin word for cow, vacca, and the process is called vaccination—a term still used today.

"Until the year 1881, long after Jenner died, the terms *vaccine* and *vaccination* were associated exclusively with the disease, smallpox. In that year, Pasteur, as a way of honoring Jenner, recommended that these terms be used to describe all such procedures that produce immunity to a disease. There are now all sorts of vaccines and vaccination procedures against diseases such as polio, measles, chickenpox, rabies, anthrax, and others, but these shouldn't trouble us this evening. It does demonstrate, however, how complicated things have become since Jenner's time.

"It is also of interest that Jenner used the term *virus* when referring to cowpox serum that he injected into the skin to produce immunity. Jenner and the early doctors, when using this word, simply meant *a specific transmission poison;* the composition of its essential qualities were unknown. Jenner had no idea that his cowpox serum contained an infective agent that we now know is a form of living matter that we call a *virus.*

"Pasteur had a great respect for Jenner, and was indebted to him for establishing some of the fundamental principles in medicine that led to the development of the sciences of bacteriology, virology and immunology."

"Professor, may I ask you something?"

"Yes, Mrs. Jones." The Prof never used a person's first name unless instructed to do so by the individual—sometimes several times. He seemed reluctant to call a person by his or her given name. Perhaps it didn't sit well with his rather formal English demeanor, which was that of a proper gentleman, at all times.

"Please, call me Valerie. I have heard so much about Lady Montagu and the role she played in the use of smallpox inoculation, during the early part of the eighteenth century. How effective was she, in her attempt to prevent smallpox disease in England?"

"First of all, let me say this, Valerie. During the eighteenth century, there were two distinct and differing ideas about how to prevent smallpox, and unless you have a clear concept of what was happening, the story could become confusing. Early in the century, smallpox inoculation was used in an attempt to prevent the disease. Later, near the end of the century, Jenner developed vaccination as a preventive measure."

"I don't mean to nag you, Professor," Valerie said, "but it seems to me Lady Montagu's story is frightfully important to the history of smallpox. Shouldn't we hear more about her?"

"Besides," interjected Ruth Goldman, the wife of Dr. Murray Goldman, the Canadian doctor on leave and also working at the Prof's laboratory, "you brought up the association of the loss of beauty and smallpox, and the ladies undoubtedly want to know more about that."

"Hear, hear!" The ladies exclaimed in unison. They were attempting to gang up on the Prof, without his realizing it.

"Well," stammered the Prof, not quite sure of himself under the circumstances. He had obviously made up his mind that the evening would be spent talking about Jenner. Any deviation from a contemplated plan was difficult for him to accept. He flinched at the thought. "Well.... I had intended to have a discussion about Dr. Jenner, this evening."

"Please, Lawrence," implored his wife, "I know that you are familiar with Lady Montagu and the part that she played in the history of smallpox, so do try to satisfy the curiosity of the rest of us. Surely you can put Dr. Jenner aside for a few minutes."

"I suppose you're right," he responded submissively. "Lady Montagu was an exciting woman who knew her own mind. Perhaps, today, she would be referred to as an activist."

"Oh, come, come, Lawrence," said Iris. Mrs. Penfield always called her husband Lawrence in the presence of company, but how she addressed him, when they were alone, is impossible to know. "Can't you see the ladies are anxious to know more about Lady Montagu. I'm sure you remember that Ruth wrote a lengthy article about Lady Montagu for a ladies' magazine, a few years back."

"You're quite right," said Prof, "maybe Ruth will fill us in on the part played by Lady Montagu in the history of smallpox. What do you say, Ruth? Will you have a go at it?"

Ruth was originally from Israel and had served in the Israeli military, in a rather important and secretive capacity, and her reticence to talk about it was understandable. After leaving Israel, she traveled widely. In fact, for a short time, she was an airline stewardess on a major international airline, that is, until she married Murray. Once she settled in Canada, she began writing short stories, often based upon her own experiences. The article that she wrote about Lady Montagu was quite by chance. It was during one of her trips to England, as an airline stewardess, that she heard mention of Lady Montagu. Subsequent remarks made about Lady Montagu's numerous exploits prompted Ruth to do some research and write an article about her for a ladies' magazine. It was during her research that Ruth discovered her subject had traveled extensively and experienced some fascinating adventures. Perhaps Lady Montagu's exploits mimicked some of her own, and it was for this reason Ruth decided to write about her.

Ruth was forty-five years old, of average height for a female, say, five feet three or four inches. She had an oval face, straight nose, and wide mouth with full lips. A head of wavy chestnut-brown hair framed her pretty eyes and flawless white skin. Her clothes were becomingly sedate and enhanced her comely appearance.

"My dear Mrs. Goldman—pardon me, Ruth," said the Prof, "before you get started, please permit me to say that in order to understand Lady Montagu and her place in the history of smallpox, I must first tell you about the disease, during the time in which she lived, which was the early part of the eighteenth century. By that time, smallpox was known and feared worldwide. Most everyone agreed that smallpox was the most dreaded disease of its time. During the seventeenth and eighteenth centuries, the disease was both cyclical, that is, it occurred in waves, and varied in its severity. When Lady Montagu lived in London, smallpox was both rampant and deadly throughout England."

Ruth finally saw her opportunity and she grasped the conversation away from the Prof; it was something few people would attempt to do.

Her husband, Murray, appeared perturbed.

She ignored him and continued, "Well, anyway, Prof, Lady Montagu championed the idea of smallpox inoculation. As you have mentioned, Prof, inoculation means the use of a form of the smallpox virus that has been weakened, after it had previously caused the disease in another person. But, first, let's go back to the beginning and develop her story.

"As a single young woman…."

◆ ◆ ◆

As a single young woman, Lady Montagu was known as Lady Mary Pierrepon, the oldest daughter of the Earl of Kingston. She was an extraordinarily beautiful and strong-minded young lady, who grew up in the luxury and leisure befitting the aristocracy of the seventeenth and eighteenth centuries. Mary's mother had died unexpectedly, when she was but fourteen years old, a calamity which she remembered to her dying day, since she was left in the sole care of her father, the Earl. Like many of the privileged class, he was "abandoned to his pleasures," and not attentive to his children's schooling. But notwithstanding some early setbacks in her education, Mary taught herself Latin grammar and other foreign languages, in order to read the works of any author she wished. With the aid of an uncommonly good memory and indefatigable energy, she gained a reputation as a scholar, a distinction not usually associated with a woman of her rank at that time.

In her late teens, during the winter social season in London, Mary attracted the attention of Edward Wortley Montagu, a gentleman somewhat senior in age to her. They had met during a festive event, and he was immediately charmed by her remarkable beauty, wit, intelligence and sagacious use of Latin, all of which belied her young age.

If Edward was apprehensive about eventually courting Mary, it was because he was eleven years older than she. In spite of what he considered an initial obstacle—the age difference—he was a handsome man with a sterling career, and he decided to curry her favor.

Mary was an especially prudent lass and was not prepared to make any commitments, knowing that she had so many wealthy and renowned admirers seeking her approval. Finally, however, Edward prevailed, but only after a most difficult and trying courtship.

All was not well for Edward, even though he convinced Mary that they should wed. Mary's father, the Earl, objected strenuously to their marriage, so much so that he refused to give Edward Mary's twenty-thousand-pound dowry. The argument over the dowry persisted for some time, it being a matter of honor for Edward and his family that the dowry be paid. Despite the Earl's intransigence, Mary and Edward decided to elope.

Nothing ever seemed to go smoothly for this loving couple, insomuch as, during the final week before their elopement, they did nothing but squabble. Mary, always so self-assured, now seemed somewhat dubious about her decision to marry Edward.

Edward, on the other hand, was more steadfast and proclaimed, "I shall wish to die with you, rather than to live without you in the highest circumstances of Fortune."

Mary, still uncertain, declared, "I tremble for what we are doing. Shall we never repent?"

Despite the continuous bickering, the couple finally eloped two days later. Mary, by then in her early twenties, henceforth was known as Lady Mary Wortley Montagu. Thirty years later, she would confide to a friend that, for a month before her marriage, she scarcely slept one night because she had such a vast number of suitors, she couldn't decide whom to choose.

In due course, Edward's career flourished in Parliament and Mary became part of London society. The union must have been blissful, since it wasn't long before Mary gave birth to her first child, a son, whom they christened Edward Wortley Montagu, Jr.

Yet no matter how satisfying the marriage, the couple would soon be tormented by the disease that everyone feared—smallpox. First, Mary was informed that her brother had fallen ill with it, and was being cared for by Doctor Garth, a highly regarded London physician and a personal friend of the Earl.

Two days after her brother developed the disease, Doctor Garth noted that the pocks were dangerously full on his face and, in less than a week, the poor man was dead. Lady Mary was grief-stricken with the loss of her closest family companion.

Still, at Court, Edward and Mary continued to enjoy an active political and social life, under the reign of a new King. By virtue of her beauty and intellectual accomplishments, Lady Mary was a favorite of the Royal family; and Edward gained influence with the King who liked to transact business speaking French, a language that Edward spoke fluently.

But pain and agony would strike the couple once again for, in little more than two years after her brother died of smallpox, Mary awoke one morning sick with a fever. Kate, her maid, touched Mary's brow and determined that she had an unusually high temperature. It wasn't long before Mary began vomiting, and became excessively drowsy and prostrate.

Kate did her best to comfort her mistress. She bathed her tenderly, to reduce her temperature, and offered her sips of water and broth to help maintain her strength. All these efforts were of little avail. Mary remained in a dazed condition throughout that day and the following night. On the second day of her illness, she developed a bright red rash over her body, most prominently over her upper thighs and buttocks; but before the day was over, the rash began to fade. In spite of this, Mary's overall condition didn't improve and even showed signs of worsening. By the time it took the doctor to arrive, Mary's rash had faded and she was now developing small raised reddish lesions on her face, arms and hands. Her early symptoms, and the appearance of the new lesions on her face, presaged a severe attack of smallpox. After a cursory history and a superficial physical examination, the doctor confirmed a diagnosis of smallpox.

The news overwhelmed Mary, since she knew what smallpox was capable of doing to her: causing disfigurement or even death. She was attended by two of the finest physicians in London, one being Doctor Garth, the same doctor who had treated her brother. Doctor Garth did what he could to cure the disease, but all was in vain. Mary eventually survived, but not without severe consequences—her beauty was marred forever. The source of her beauty, her delicate facial skin, was deeply pitted and she was left without eyelashes. Soon after she recovered, Mary expressed the terror and trepidation that she experienced, during her bout with smallpox, in poems that she penned and sent to friends.

Within a year after her illness, Edward was appointed Ambassador Extraordinary to the Court of Turkey. It was a prestigious appointment for Edward, and for Lady Mary it was to be an event that would bring her everlasting fame and change the way smallpox was treated in England.

Preparations for such an extensive journey of unknown duration required careful planning. Aside from the household things and personal items of clothing that had to be packed, Mary had to decide which of the servants would accompany them. She debated with herself about taking her son on such a long and dangerous journey; finally, however, she settled on taking the child and a nurse to care for him.

Their route to Turkey was another contentious issue, but it was eventually determined that they should go by way of Vienna, so that Edward could deliver a message to the Emperor. With that settled, the family embarked on a private yacht at Gravesend, early in August of 1717. The trip, however, was not without incident. The yacht, which was headed for a port in Holland, was soon becalmed for two days, and to add to their misfortune, it was afterwards battered by a severe storm. To Mary, the captain appeared alarmed, but not Mary, for later she was to boast that she "neither felt fear nor sea-sickness."

As their entourage of carriages traveled to the various western European capitals, Edward and Mary were entertained as royalty, because of the prestigious appointment that he held. For Mary, this was a new and a pleasing experience. Still, the journey was not without its complications, but in spite of the labyrinth in which she was involved, she loved every moment of her new adventure. Always keen to learn, Mary made good use of her newly gained knowledge. For example, while being entertained in the king's palace, one evening during the cold of December, she was served oranges, lemons and pineapples. What made all this possible were the plain stoves that her host had devised, to maintain the proper growing temperature for the plants and trees in his plant-houses. Highly decorated versions of these same stoves were used to warm the rooms in his palatial home. Mary was impressed and made a mental note to use this information, when the opportunity presented itself. She realized that there was no need to freeze in London, during the cold winter months, so when she returned home, she had one of these stoves placed in each of the home's sleeping chambers.

Fortunately, the winter was mild and their coaches and sleighs traveled easily and swiftly through the snow. Throughout the early part of the journey, their entourage was accompanied by a few royal guards but, as they approached Turkey, diplomatic protocol became more ostentatious, with 200 soldiers replacing the royal guards. At the border, the soldiers were relieved, and the party was escorted by 130 Turkish guards on horseback.

While Edward was waiting to be summoned by the Sultan to Adrianople, a city outside of Constantinople, they were given a deluxe and ornate apartment. By this time, the group had been traveling for six months and Mary welcomed the respite, and she used the delay wisely. It was her first exposure to the two divergent sides of the Turkish culture: an opulent life-style versus despotic barbarism. What she enjoyed most was the Arabian poetry with its musical measures, and she reacted most favorably to the romantic poetry, because it was passionate and lively.

After three weeks, Edward was summoned to move on to his final destination, Adrianople. It was Mary's first encounter with one of the hidden dangers of the East: the plague. In the course of the journey one of her servants became ill, and though he eventually survived, he was diagnosed as having had the dreaded scourge.

During their trip to Adrianople, they stopped to visit one of the famous hot Turkish baths. Mary relates how, incognito, she slipped away from her companions to experience the Turkish form of female bathing. Later, she described the charming female bathers who, having seen her corseted, thought that she had been locked in the garment by a jealous husband.

Once they arrived in Adrianople, Mary lived in a palace provided by the Sultan for her husband, the new Ambassador. Mary's facility for languages enabled her to quickly learn enough Turkish to travel alone, disguised in a local Turkish costume. Her regional costume, consisting of loose, full robes and heavy veil, buried her true identity. The costume served its intended purpose, since it enabled her to visit sites otherwise restricted to most Europeans.

In the course of one of her solitary outings she, for the first time, saw the practice of smallpox inoculation. The procedure previously had been described in the 1714 and 1716 Transactions of the Royal Society in London, but they were mainly ignored by the English physicians. After watching the procedure performed many times and learning more about it from the local physicians, Mary judged smallpox inoculation to be simple and safe, and she was determined to have it done on her son as soon as practicable. Being a visionary, she realized that if the practice of smallpox inoculation could be introduced in her country, England, it would help to control the disease and eliminate a lot of unnecessary suffering. Her enthusiasm for smallpox inoculation was directly related to her own terrifying experience with the disease, a few years previously. As an example of her zeal, she wrote the following sentence in a letter to a friend in London:

"I am patriot enough to take pains to bring this useful invention into fashion in England; and I should not fail to write to some of our doctors very particularly about it."

This promise was no hollow boast, but a model for her future behavior.

Even though she was pregnant with her second child, Mary continued to write and to participate in the varied activities at the Sultan's court. In February of 1718, she gave birth to a girl. Mary received the best of care, during her pregnancy and delivery by Doctor Maitland, the Embassy surgeon, and Doctor Emanuel Timoni, an eminent Constantinople physician. It was the same Doctor Timoni who first described smallpox inoculation in the records of the Royal Society, in 1714. In addition, he was able to persuade her to have her son inoculated against smallpox.

Once convinced of the safety of smallpox inoculation, Mary agreed to have her six-year-old son inoculated. A suitable person from whom to extract the smallpox matter was found by Dr. Maitland. After this, an old Greek woman, who practiced smallpox inoculation for many years, inoculated the child. The doctor describes how the old woman's hands were shaking, as she scratched the smallpox material into the skin of the boy's arm with a blunt, rusted needle. During the procedure, the boy was in constant pain, so much so, that Doctor Maitland decided to inoculate the child's other arm himself.

"I pitied his cries and, therefore, Inoculated the other arm with my own Instruments, and with so little pain to him, that he did not in the least complain of it."

Fortunately, for the child, he developed only a mild case of smallpox and was never in danger. On the third day, he developed a fever and a spotted rash on his face. By the eighth day, multiple pustules were present on his face; however, they crusted and dropped off without scarring. Minor scars on both of his arms, at the sites of inoculation, were the only evidence of the operation.

Mary deferred from having her daughter inoculated with smallpox, since the child's nurse never had the disease and would be in danger of contracting it from the child, once the little girl was inoculated.

After two years of foreign service, Edward and his family were back in London where he served the remainder of his life in Parliament. Upon her return to London, Mary resumed the place in society that she held before leaving for Turkey. Thus, she was able, by her privileged position, to advance the cause of smallpox inoculation.

In the spring of 1721, there was a vicious smallpox epidemic present in London. For whatever reason, the fatality rate among children was particularly high. Fortunately, through Mary's exhaustive efforts, public interest in smallpox inoculation was increasing rapidly. It also helped that many London physicians began doing smallpox inoculations, in addition to issuing pamphlets promoting the procedure.

It was at this time that Lady Mary solicited Doctor Maitland, now living in England, to inoculate her daughter. Without the usual preparatory ritual of bleeding and purging, Doctor Maitland scratched the weakened smallpox matter into the skin on both arms of the child. Three members of the College of Physicians were permitted to visit the child at different times, their purpose being to certify that the child was doing well, following the inoculation. With a flare for the dramatic, Lady Mary also verified the child's excellent health and her belief that "a miracle had occurred."

Only after Lady Mary had her daughter successfully inoculated with smallpox, was she able to convince members of the Royal Family and the Court to have smallpox inoculation performed on their children. The Princess Caroline was the first to try inoculation. She had her two daughters inoculated with the smallpox matter, but only after she first had the procedure performed on criminals and orphans. Once members of the Royal Family had their own children inoculated, and only then, was smallpox inoculation adopted for use by the general public.

The extreme dangers of smallpox inoculation were recognized, only after the procedure was widely used and accepted by the general public, which is frequently the case with newly used medical discoveries. Some of the inoculated children died; others lived but were left with the hideous scars of the disease; and generalized epidemics of smallpox occurred in communities where children recently had been inoculated.

Still, many children and adults were successfully inoculated without problems occurring, and it can be safely said that the procedure saved lives.

While smallpox inoculation eventually became extensively used throughout England, still there were those among both the physicians and clergy who condemned its use. In fact, some countries prohibited the procedure altogether, for fear that those being inoculated would spread the disease to members of the population who never had the disease, and in this way start an epidemic—which is exactly what sometimes occurred. Nonetheless, Lady Mary Montagu continued to be extensively eulogized, in pamphlets supporting smallpox inoculation, for bringing the procedure to England. Her name continues to be associated with smallpox inoculation, long after the procedure has been replaced by vaccination, developed by Dr. Edward Jenner, in the latter part of the eighteenth century.

5

NOW THAT LADY MONTAGU had been discussed to the satisfaction of the wives, Prof directed his remarks to the disease itself and its consequences. "Murray, except for smallpox, your country, Canada, would likely now to be just another state of your southern neighbor, the United States of America."

Dr. Goldman fumbled and fumed at the aspersion that Canada might have become a part of the United States. Such an unbelievable remark! Once Murray regained his composure, he came to the defense of his country, with mellow-toned comments that masked his umbrage at the Prof's remarks. He knew that he was being confronted by two formidable opponents: an indefatigable English professor and a super-patriotic American doctor. Murray decided that he would proceed with caution, so he said, "I'm not sure that most Canadians would agree, Prof, but I'm willing to listen to the premise of your argument."

But it was Dr. Jones, known informally as Jimmy to the group, who defended the argument that Canada would now be part of the United States, if it hadn't been for an outbreak of smallpox among the American soldiers that stopped their conquest of Eastern Canada, in 1775.

Jimmy was a good-looking fellow who proved to be an ideal collaborator and assistant to the Professor in his laboratory. Ordinarily quiet and easygoing, he did not hesitate to make his point in a discussion or argument. Jimmy had a short nose and well formed mouth with strong, white teeth that seemed to stare at you when he smiled—which was often. He had wavy black hair and thick eyebrows which contrasted well with his soft blue eyes. Jimmy was in his mid-forties, six feet tall, strongly built and well proportioned, undoubtedly characteristics that he inherited from his Irish ancestors.

A well respected faculty member of the prestigious mid-west University of Chicago, Jimmy was studying advanced biology and mathematics with the Prof. He and his wife and children had already been in London for two years. They loved the city and were just now becoming comfortable with some of the unusual English customs. In Chicago, his family was both highly respected and wealthy. It was Jimmy's father who improvised and contrived ways to give the family the desired air of respectability, but it was his Irish immigrant grandfather who made all the money that, one day, would enable the family to become financial and social leaders in the area. Good, old grandpa was tough as nails and saved his money but, underneath the polished veneer, grandpa was still shanty Irish. Grandma had been a German housekeeper to a respectable Chicago family. Grandma, too, immigrated to Chicago, arriving there shortly before grandpa. The old girl had very little formal education, but she was naturally intelligent and observant. Once she was settled into her housekeeper position, she quickly learned to speak and write proper English, which she was determined to speak without a German accent. Old granny was inquisitive and an avid reader. The home of her employers had an extensive library, and every evening and on her days off, she spent her time reading about many subjects. Grandma was fascinated by the family's dinner conversations, which she overheard, as she served the meals. The discussions eventually turned to finances and the stock market. Grandma soon realized that she had to read and learn more about investing, if she were to become financially secure. She observed and assimilated the dignified manners of the family and, by the time she left their employment, years later, she had a substantial bank account and the manners and grace of a socially respectable young lady.

After grandpa and grandma married, they combined his desire for wealth with her knowledge of economics and the stock market, to eventually amass a small fortune. It was grandma who taught Jimmy the qualities that are the marks of a cultured gentleman—and it was grandpa who gave the University of Chicago a few million dollars, to educate his son and grandson.

Ambitious and eager to make a contribution to science, Jimmy arranged to join Prof's staff for two years. He could have led the life of a Chicago playboy, spending grandpa's hard-earned money, as his older brother was wont to do. Jimmy, however, was altruistic; he wanted to add something to life and not just take from it.

The Jones family enjoyed their stay in London and not once had they talked about leaving. The cultural and social life of London was so cosmopolitan and exciting that they wanted to make the most of it. For Jimmy, the laboratory experience was all that he could ask for.

The three Jones children, ages 6 thru 14, a boy and two girls, enjoyed attending their English schools. They found the classwork was well organized and the students were more respectful of their teachers than was usually the case back home in Chicago. Life in their American schools was becoming disorganized and disorderly. While the discipline was much stricter in the English schools, the children welcomed the orderliness, as it made their classwork more enjoyable and enhanced their ability to learn.

But life in England was more than schoolwork for the Jones brood. There were family weekend outings to castles and historical places; and outdoor lunches that Valerie prepared for the family to enjoy, as they sat up in the green hills watching gliders being towed for take-off by a propeller-driven plane. Once aloft, the gliders were released and they soared back and forth overhead, soundlessly and seemingly effortlessly, for long periods of time, on the shoulders of the wind. On special weekends, the family attended plays in the wonderful, old, downtown London theatres. And during the summer vacations, they camped out, while touring Europe. But their very special summer vacation was to take an overnight ship from the great port of Liverpool, famous for commerce of men and material between England and Ireland, and cross the wild Irish Sea to Belfast, Northern Ireland. From there the family drove their station wagon to the northwest coastal town of

Donegal, which is part of the Irish Free State and the place from which their great-grandfather had originated. Oh, how happy they were to find their roots, to visit their great-grandmother's old, thatched-roof farmhouse, and to walk in the hills that overlooked the turbulent Atlantic Ocean below. They just knew that if they could see past the horizon, there would be an unobstructed view of America.

The past two years had been full of many happy days for the family. Jimmy and Valerie were somewhat saddened that one day soon they would have to leave all of it, but later—not just yet.

Jimmy was anxious to defend the States and to advance the Prof's thesis that except for the disease, smallpox, Canada would now be part of the United States.

"Prof," said Dr. Jones, "the story begins early on in our War of Independence...."

◆   ◆   ◆

From the start of The American War of Independence, or as it is sometimes referred to by the English, The American Revolutionary War, all sorts of diseases plagued General Washington's ill equipped army. However, the disease that was most feared, and the greatest killer of them all was smallpox. It could spread rapidly through the ranks, and kill a quarter of the troops but, worst of all, it could debilitate large numbers of soldiers at the time of a critical battle. General Washington knew this, as did Napoleon at a later time in the century.

In July 1775, General Washington was headquartered outside Boston. The Battle of Bunker Hill, one of the battles that started the war, was now nine months past, and still Washington's command was nothing but a skeleton, a facade of a real army. The Army must act, and its most obvious opponents were the English forces in possession of nearby Boston. But an epidemic of smallpox was occurring there, and Washington feared the disease more than he dreaded the English guns and cannons.

After the battles at Lexington and Concord, General Washington ordered all English prisoners to be guarded by those of his troops who already had had smallpox. He reasoned that since the English used smallpox against the Indians, during their westerly campaigns, they would do the same thing against his army, whose men were as vulnerable to the disease as were the Indians.

The smallpox epidemic was carried into the city by the refugees flooding the area. Washington was at a tactical disadvantage, and he knew it. General Howe's English troops were less prone to contract smallpox than were his own, since the majority of English soldiers either had the disease naturally, as children, or were given it by inoculation, as was the custom in the army at that time. On the other hand, Washington's colonial troops, fresh from the countryside, having never been exposed to the disease, were much more susceptible to it. Washington, therefore, was apprehensive and aware of what the dreaded smallpox could do to his troops.

The so-called war now taking place was extraordinary, to say the least. Instead of attempting to destroy each other with bullets and cannonballs, the two opposing armies were attempting do it with a disease—smallpox.

Washington had suspected that Howe was purposefully forcing smallpox victims to leave Boston and intermingle with the other refugees, in hopes of infecting Washington's soldiers. As a means of protecting his army from smallpox, Washington had all the refugees leaving Boston inspected and thoroughly fumigated, in an attempt to prevent them from contaminating the troops. And so the war was fought, in its early stages, one army endeavoring to overwhelm the other with smallpox.

In July of 1775, Washington complained to Congress, expressing his concern about his troops being exposed to smallpox. In the letter he said, "I have been particularly attentive to the least symptom of the smallpox, and hitherto we have been so fortunate as to have every person removed, so soon as noting, to prevent any communication, but I am apprehensive it may gain in the camps. We shall continue the utmost vigilance against this most dangerous enemy."

For Washington, smallpox was a real threat; he knew how easily this disease could lay waste to his small ragtag army. Smallpox was not new to him; he had contracted it while visiting Barbados in 1751. His pockmarked face was testimony to his having survived his battle with a most vicious foe. Uppermost on Washington's mind was how to prevent losing the war to smallpox, before the real battles were even fought.

Regardless of his vigilance, Washington was unable to shield his men from contracting the disease, so new cases occurred daily. Together with the bloody flux—some said from drinking raw cider—sickness was rapidly depleting Washington's ranks.

Each morning, Washington dressed in his blue and buff uniform, with a blue ribbon across his chest designating that he was the Commanding General. Along with his staff officers, some as young as 18 years of age, he inspected the poorly trained soldiers making up his people's army. This do-nothing-army was weary—as were Washington and Congress. The men began complaining about incessant drilling and "no action." The enemy, the English army, could be seen in Boston by the Charles River, waiting for an attack by Washington's army that never came.

Washington's Staff Meeting:

"Sir, how much longer can we remain here before we attack Boston? Each day we are losing men to sickness, and those who are healthy want to fight and go home," said his Chief of Staff. The rest of the officers either nodded in agreement or said, "Aye."

Washington, noted for his taciturnity, said nothing but stared straight ahead reflecting, as if he hadn't heard the question. He was thinking about his poorly trained soldiers, his limited supply of powder and artillery, and his need for the additional men that Congress had promised him. The colonies, with a population of over two million, surely could find additional troops to enable him to attack the British, with a force twice their size.

Washington decided to break the silence and said, "Gentlemen, we are going to attack—not Boston, as you wish, but Canada."

The silence was deadly. For a moment no one spoke, when suddenly, in unison they all cried, "Canada?" almost in disbelief.

In the small huts and tents of the soldiers, the word "Canada" circulated as rapidly as did the location of the local prostitutes' nests. Each soldier had his own comment, but the one heard most often was, "Canada! Why Canada? Boston is nearer."

An in-the-know sergeant, who got his information firsthand from a reputedly reliable source, said, "Washington fears that British troops in Canada are about to move south to divide New England from the rest of the Colonies." While this short summation of Washington's strategy may have been partially true, the reasons for invading Canada were more complex than that.

Two of Washington's outspoken and aggressive confidants, Benedict Arnold and Ethan Allen, argued in favor of an invasion of Canada, which, if successful, would confirm Washington's military superiority as a General and as a leader of men. At the same time, it would incorporate the Canadian territories into the union as a fourteenth colony. Their arguments favoring an invasion of Canada—most favored the euphemism "liberate," rather than "invasion"—were both political and religious. Washington finally agreed that Allen would join in an attack on Montreal, and Colonel Arnold would lead a force of 1,100 soldiers via the Kennebeck River, using bateaux—flat-bottom boats—and attack Quebec. Both of these military operations were difficult, incurring many obstacles, and essentially were destined for failure, but for reasons other than just military incompetence.

Washington had to move quickly with his plans for the invasion, since his militant rebels, once aching for a fight, were now bored from hanging around for over half a year. Some soldiers were deserting to return to their farms and care for their crops; others had grown weary;

many were sick and debilitated, principally with smallpox, since it was constantly present throughout the encampment. By the end of the year 1775, only half of Washington's more than four thousand troops stationed on Prospect Hill were fit to fight.

When enlistments expired, troops disregarded the pleas of their officers and simply left. The "spirit of '76" was already on the decline during the second half of '75.

At this critical time, Washington asked for volunteers for an expedition to liberate Canada. The liberation was the sort of adventure that appealed to the young, adventurous soldiers in his army. Eleven hundred fidgety soldiers volunteered to takes flat-bottom boats through the Maine wilderness and liberate Quebec, which was to be the first major offensive by the American army during the war.

The officer-in-command of the expedition was Colonel Benedict Arnold, who had previously captured Fort Ticonderoga from the British. Later in the war, he would become known as a famous traitor to the American cause. Lieutenant Colonel Roger Enos was under Arnold's command, and he, too, would turn out to be a military misfit.

While Arnold and Enos were brave fighters, they lacked the one quality that Napoleon considered essential for all successful leaders, namely an element of luck. Napoleon believed that one either had this quality about them or they did not; it wasn't a trait that one could deliberately attempt to cultivate or to feign. Neither Arnold nor Enos was "lucky;" Smallpox would decimate their troops on the way to Canada, and it would decide the day for the British army.

Still, many of the troops kept asking, "Why Canada of all places?" No one seemed quite sure. It is difficult to know how an invasion of a foreign colony was linked to the problems faced at home. Some say Washington wanted to prevent the British troops in Quebec from moving south and cutting off the New England colonies from the main body of his troops surrounding Boston. Perhaps, but the Yankees, mostly fervent Protestants, were easily motivated to attack the citadel of Catholicism on their northern border. For the Yankee

Protestant, there was a similarity between the political tyranny of the British monarch and the religious absolutism of the Pope. Therefore, a continental purging for political and religious reasons held the promise of removing both tyrants at once.

Whatever Washington's reason for attacking Quebec, the expedition was a tactical misadventure.

Colonel Arnold, tall and bulky, in his middle thirties, spoke with his newly formed army, hoping to energize them in this new crusade. If the truth were known, Arnold always wanted to invade Canada, especially after he had captured Fort Ticonderoga, but he was stopped from doing so by the officers and officials of Massachusetts—whom he never forgave.

The plan was simple: General Schuyler would leave Fort Ticonderoga and attack Montreal in Canada; and after he completed the capture of Montreal, his troops would then join Arnold, and jointly they would attack Quebec. American spies assured Arnold there was no British fleet and only seven hundred troops guarding Quebec. Had his troops remained healthy, Arnold easily could have defeated such a small British garrison. In addition, Arnold was assured, mistakenly, that the Canadians would welcome him and desert their English allies. While the truth of the matter was that the Canadians, especially the French Canadians, disliked the English, they distrusted their American neighbors even more. The French Canadians were well aware of the Americans' bitterness towards the Roman Catholic Church in French Canada. Arnold and Washington were foolish to assume that the French Canadians would welcome their troops, knowing the animosity the American Protestants had for their church.

Arnold's army proceeded to the mouth of the Kennebec River where they boarded 224 bateaux—wooden flat-bottom boats. The plan was to travel up the Kennebec River to the Canadian border where they would enter the Chaudiere River and proceed on to Quebec. As this military force would come to know, navigating the flat-bottom boats up rivers, against swift currents, presented many unanticipated problems and obstacles. The men rowed, and at times, had to drag the boats; in places, they even abandoned the river and portaged the boats over distances as much as several miles. Just getting to Quebec was such a struggle that it weakened both the men and the boats. Some of the men drowned, when the damaged boats sank in the river. The troops had difficulty remaining dry, as their small boats floundered in the river, fighting the swift currents; but worst of all, the men had difficulty keeping their powder dry, as they forded the many streams. Fall, with its foul weather, had already arrived as they departed from Boston, and soon cold, wet weather and snow were to plague them as they advanced. Partway into their journey, their food was used up, so they had to forage in order to keep alive. Soon, to add to their misery, men began coming down with smallpox.

Washington's greatest fear was now realized: some of the men under Arnold's command had contracted smallpox before leaving Boston.

As Arnold's command moved ever farther northward, more and more of his men became feverish and weak, eventually showing telltale spots of smallpox. Those infected had to remain where they were, since they were too weak to travel. A quarter of the infected soldiers died, while there were many others, who were not sick, but refused to continue on with the expedition for fear of getting the disease. Those who were ill, and had been left in the woods, probably died pondering the meaning of life, and also questioning whether or not the journey was really worth it. Those soldiers, with strength to return home, questioned whether their problem with the King was worth the sacrifices they had made.

As one of Arnold's officers observed, "As fine an army as ever marched into Canada has to be entirely ruined by the dreaded smallpox."

Early in November 1775, Arnold gathered his ragtag army at a point on the St. Lawrence River across from Quebec. Before reaching this position, Arnold received word that the feckless Lieutenant Colonel Enos had deserted with his troops and returned to Massachusetts.

The desertions, and the deaths caused by smallpox in Arnold's army, reduced their number from the original eleven hundred men to five hundred now facing fortress Quebec.

Arnold laid siege to Quebec, but was unable to attack the city. His army's ranks had been depleted by disease, and much of his ammunition and supplies had been lost or rendered useless, in the course of the trip through Maine. Arnold delayed attacking the city, until General Montgomery arrived with three hundred additional men and much needed military supplies.

This delay would prove costly, because Arnold's ranks continued to be depleted by the dreaded smallpox, while the English were able to use the time to organize their forces in the defense of the city.

When the attack took place on New Year's Eve, nature, in the form of a snowstorm, added to the difficulties which led to the defeat of Arnold and his brave men. Arnold was wounded and General Montgomery was killed, as they led their men in the first charge on the city. Still, Arnold's men were unyielding, as they scaled the walls of the city and entered the lower town but, unfortunately, Montgomery's men failed to come to their aid. In the end, Arnold's men were surrounded and captured.

That night, over four hundred American soldiers were taken prisoner. For a half year, they were imprisoned under the worst of conditions, and many of them died of smallpox. Those who survived were set free by the English General Carleton, after they signed a paper promising to "lay at home & no come to trouble him."

Later, John Adams would write, "Smallpox was ten times more terrible than Britons, Canadians and Indians together."

After the war was over, some would say that smallpox, in all probability, was the worst killer of the Revolution.

◆   ◆   ◆

"You're right, Jim," said the Professor, still sipping his wine. "The terrifying smallpox plagued the colonies, in 1775, and lasted as long as the Revolutionary War—until 1782. Eventually, the entire country was infected with smallpox. Whereas the Revolutionary War politically characterized the eighteenth century for the Americans, during that same time, smallpox was the disease that brought misery and suffering to the entire American continent."

6

WITHOUT REALIZING WHAT WAS HAPPENING, ALL THE guests, as well as the Prof and his wife, were themselves being inextricably woven into the story. An evening designated for rest, recreation and relaxation was slowly and surely changing, as the storytellers were tantalized and tormented in their efforts to tell the tale honestly.

Professor Penfield sensed the tenor and tone of the discussions were now more directed and intense. It was as if, as the participants spoke, they were personally and irrevocably becoming part of the story. Conceivably, the old, mysterious house, with its hidden underground vault and its secret panel in the wall of the master bedroom—where the priest was hidden from that vindictive old tyrant, Oliver Cromwell, and his "Round Heads"—was using its magic to transport the guests to another time and place.

The Prof always maintained that the house was haunted; that it was preyed upon by some unearthly spirits which affected people's behavior and thinking. When and how these things occurred he didn't know, but they surely happened in the minds of the children and the Prof. Everything he told them was all very real on account of the fact that they could see it all in their minds, as if it were a movie. Unfortunately, the adults long ago lost this wonderful ability of seeing mind-pictures—all adults except the Prof, of course. The children just loved hearing the same stories over and over again, and they never seemed to tire of them. It was, perhaps, because they had such active and vivid imaginations that their mind-pictures changed each time they heard the same story retold. The Prof knew this, and he used it to his advantage. Conceivably, his mind-pictures also changed each time he repeated one of his stories.

Occasionally, during the daylight hours, he escorted the guests' children through the dark and dreary corridors into the many elephantine rooms with their secret hiding places, foreboding, dark, wood-paneled walls and old-fashioned, overstuffed furniture. As he led his parade of anxious and inquisitive youngsters, he described for them, in fearsome detail, those individuals who had died in the beds in each of the rooms. To lower the veil of mystery even more, and stimulate the imagination and excitement of his attentive listeners, he told them about the people who were mysteriously murdered in some of those same beds. But of all the fascinating and tantalizing rooms in the old house, it was the cell-like vault in the basement, referred to affectionately as the "dungeon" by the children, which was by far their favorite room. Who knows why they so loved the dungeon. Maybe that room challenged their vivid imaginations to conjure up strange events that might have taken place there, centuries ago. Of course, in the minds of the children, all ancient ordeals were horrible, for how else could the dungeon be so frightening? No matter how spooky that jail-like chamber was, it was the place that they loved best to visit—but never alone.

After one of these tours, which the children looked forward to, whenever they visited Prof, the first thing the children did was run to find their parents and tell them about the wonderful experience and the many stories the Prof had told them. His stories always had a funny or happy ending, even if the background in which they were told was a bit spooky. The children always assured their parents that they knew the Prof's stories were "make-believe," but the parents shouldn't tell the Prof that they knew, for he may be disappointed.

There was no doubt that the old house had somehow affected the adult guests and their thinking, too. It was as if they could not shake off the vivid description of smallpox read to them by Prof from Emile Zola's "Nana." The changes that were taking place in his guests weren't new to the Prof and Iris. They had known it to happen before in that imposing living room, when classical or historical subjects were discussed. Notwithstanding this, the Prof was anxious to press on with the Jenner story.

For a moment, he stood silently by the fireplace with its mesmerizing flames burning brightly behind him, and stared off into space. Suddenly he began rubbing his chin, and the guests then knew the storytelling was about to resume. "Cedric," he said, addressing his remarks to Professor Foxworth, "So far, this evening, I've heard about what the smallpox does to people but, on the other hand, we seem to know very little about the smallpox virus itself. Is that true?"

As soon as Cedric heard his name mentioned, he became alert and attentive. "Prof, I should love to answer your question," he said.

Everyone subconsciously addressed the Prof by his proper academic rank, Professor, except of course, at social occasions, such as this evening. Never was he referred to only by his first or last name by any of his staff, or for that matter, by any member of the university faculty of equal rank.

Cedric Foxworth had a brilliant mind and an established international-scientific reputation of his own, aside from his being in the Prof's department. He was in his mid-fifties, of average height and had a cadaverous appearance. His eyes, by contrast, were large, luminous and protruding, covered by thick horn-rimmed glasses that only exaggerated their size even more. His thin lips were pallid, as was his complexion. The nose and chin were of no interest, but his hair was not easily forgotten. He had a full head of grey hair with a softness and tenuity that seemed to have never collided with a comb or a brush; his hair appeared to naturally defy gravity. One was struck by an inconsistency in his mannerisms which contrasted with his creative, coherent, comprehensible, proper English speech.

During World War II Cedric wasn't in the military service, but functioned as a research scientist at a plant where fighter aircraft were designed. He was under great strain to keep up with the needs of the military and, eventually, suffered a complete mental and physical collapse. This episode was indicative of his high-strung nature and probably explained some of his unusual behavior and lack of sensitivity, later on in his life.

"*Tout de suite,* straightaway," Cedric responded. He was a colossal snob and used French expressions whenever possible, even when not called for. His English contemporaries in science looked askance at his hoity-toity behavior, but were willing to accept his eccentricities as long as he was able to advance the cause of science. Nor was he bashful or withdrawn, for he immediately picked-up on the discussion.

"Prof, you're correct. During Jenner's time there was no such thing as a virus, as the term is presently used, and for that matter, neither was anything known about bacteria. Jenner used the word *virus* according to its eighteenth century meaning, when referring to smallpox; that is, something corrupt or poisonous; more precisely, an evil or harmful influence. The word virus is a very old term, derived from the Latin, meaning a slimy liquid or a poison, and it was this definition that was still being used by Jenner and his peers.

"Today, virus means an ultramicroscopic particle of nucleic acid, either RNA or DNA, encased in a protein, but numerous discoveries had to be made before settling on this final description. First and foremost, were the discoveries of the great French scientist, Louis Pasteur, in the mid-nineteenth century, when he reasoned that a virus was a living particle and not a slimy liquid or a poison of evil or harmful influence. He used some of the ideas proposed by Dr. Jenner, when he developed his (virus) vaccine against rabies. Pasteur gave abundant credit to Jenner for his pioneering work with cowpox.

"In the mid-nineteen thirties, the electron microscope came into use in the field of biological research, and it was then that the smallpox virus was seen for the first time as a brick-shaped ultramicroscopic particle. More recently, using biochemical techniques, the chemical structure of the smallpox virus was identified. From this type of information, we know that the smallpox virus is complex and doesn't mutate—change its form easily."

Cedric stopped talking, took a long breath, and, in a rare moment—for him, that is—decided to act magnanimous. "Prof, you know that Jenner had none of this advanced scientific knowledge, and still he was able to reason correctly about the relationship of the disease cowpox to smallpox. He also knew that there were other pox diseases in animals that were, in some way, connected immunologically to cowpox and smallpox. He even predicted that, some day, vaccination would eliminate the disease smallpox from our planet. Quite a prediction, wouldn't you say? It shows that Jenner had a far greater knowledge of how vaccination worked in preventing smallpox than some people gave him credit for.

"His prediction that smallpox would be eliminated from our planet has theoretically happened, but it didn't occur for another two and half centuries. He was correct, nevertheless, and he deserves recognition."

Cedric again paused, appeared pensive, and said, "Sure makes you feel humble doesn't it, Prof?"

No one in the room actually believed that Cedric was capable of feeling humble. Rather, he was using one of his many little ploys to draw attention to himself and deny Jenner a victory.

"Fine, Cedric, then tell me where this virus originated," the Prof directed, as he drew a nearby chair closer to the hearth and sat down.

"Well, Prof, speculation about the origin of the disease suggests that while the exact..."

◆ ◆ ◆

While the exact origin of the smallpox virus is unknown, there is evidence that it probably had its origins as an animal poxvirus in Central Africa. Millions of years ago an animal poxvirus—and there are many of them—produced mild sickness in its primitive animal hosts. Then, sometime in its history, the virus mutated, that is, changed its chemical framework, enabling it to infect people. The disease that it produced in man was named smallpox, and it caused a severe illness which ended either in death or permanent immunity.

It would seem that smallpox has been producing pestilence in humans for quite a while. As an example, ancient Egyptian writings, over six thousand years old, suggest that smallpox was known to them. Besides, when the mummy of Ramses V, 1157 B. C., was examined, in more recent times, it showed skin lesions suggestive of the disease. Notwithstanding these findings, early medical literature had trouble identifying smallpox epidemics, since they were frequently confused with epidemics of measles. Finally, in the tenth century, a Persian-born physician living in Baghdad determined, on examination, how to distinguish smallpox from measles. From that time on, there was better reporting on smallpox epidemics.

Probably, during the early middle ages, smallpox was brought into Europe by the Crusaders on their return from the Holy Land, where smallpox was recurrent. Later, it was imported into Southern Spain during the Moorish conquest.

And for centuries, neither prince nor pauper was spared the devastating disablement of the disease. In spite of their regal surroundings, all the Royal Families of Europe had someone die, or become scarred or blinded by smallpox. Among the royalty of England, it was known as the most terrible of all the ministers of death.

Without warning, during the seventeenth and eighteenth centuries, smallpox began to have terrible repercussions on all European societies. Deaths in Europe, during these centuries, were estimated to be in the hundreds of thousands, with most of the deaths occurring in children. Deaths occurring with this intensity prevented population growth from taking place, in many of the larger cities of Europe. In the developing industrial cities of England, in order not to fall behind, immigration was needed to maintain the work force.

It is judged that smallpox killed more people than any other disease; perhaps three hundred million people have died, while millions who survived the disease were left scarred or blind. Of the two diseases, plague and smallpox, the latter was feared the most. While plague killed its victims quickly, perhaps within hours or days, smallpox produced a slow and cruel death; the process of dying could take as long as ten to sixteen days, during which time there was considerable pain and suffering. The people not only dreaded dying, but if they survived, they feared the ravages of the disease: scarring, deformity and blindness.

The plague was very different from smallpox in another important way. Plague was not that common, perhaps occurring only once or twice during the average person's lifetime. Smallpox, however, was always present and its results were forever filling the graveyards of Europe. It is no wonder, then, that anyone not yet stricken with the disease was tormented and in constant fear.

Smallpox could be a loathsome and disgusting disease, because, as the pox lesions ruptured, they became secondarily infected by bacteria, producing the foul odor of death associated with that of the rotting flesh. The odor was nauseating, and the offending stench made it difficult for those caring for the patients. Once the pustules began flowing together, survival was rare, but if a patient managed to survive this horrific ordeal, scabs formed, encrusting a major portion of the body, making movement both difficult and painful. Usually, on about the fifteenth day of suffering, the crusts separated and fell off, leaving behind whitish skin covered by repulsive pitted scars.

Smallpox was spread from lesions in the mouth and throat that exuded enormous numbers of virus particles in the saliva; therefore, the disease was passed on to others through talking, coughing or sneezing. It was the inhalation of the virus particles that produced the disease in other defenseless individuals.

7

AT THAT POINT, THE PROF DECIDED that the group should discuss Jenner's childhood. "By now, I would guess we are all agreed that smallpox is one of the world's most alarming and treacherous diseases. Yet, what do we know about Dr. Edward Jenner, the man whose discovery finally brought it under control?" The question wasn't directed at anyone in particular; however, since Cedric was an Englishman and, therefore, was supposedly knowledgeable about Dr. Jenner, he was the first to volunteer an answer.

Before replying, Cedric sat quietly, mentally crafting the words he would use.

"Get on with it, Cedric, this is not a grammatical quiz; tell us what you know about Jenner. What was he like as a young boy, and how did living in the eighteenth century, in a small, country village, influence him as an adult? Perhaps, knowing these things will enable us to better understand how it was that he was able to make his wonderful discovery that eventually led to the prevention of smallpox. We'll decide later why it was that he succeeded in accomplishing so much. Remember, others before him had heard the stories that having had cowpox would prevent an individual from contracting smallpox, and they considered these stories merely 'old wives' tales.' In settling the issue, Jenner, instead, approached the question scientifically, by gathering firsthand information from people who had had cowpox; examining the udders of cow's with disease; and, finally, vaccinating a healthy boy with cowpox and then challenging him with smallpox inoculation. But, we're getting ahead of our story. Let's go back to the beginning," the Prof said impatiently.

"Well, let's see, Jenner was born into an educated family that was well-off but not rich." Cedric paused, adjusted his eyeglasses, and then continued, "He was the youngest child in the family, being born in the middle of the eighteenth century, on May 17^{th,} 1749. Jenner was fortunate to be born in the eighteenth century, since it was a time when the rigid thinking and behavior of the sixteenth and seventeenth centuries were being cast off and a new, more progressive era was just beginning."

Ruth Goldman enthusiastically endorsed Cedric's remarks. Prompted by her interest in art and architecture she added, "The middle of the eighteenth century was the end of the Baroque period in music, art and architecture. Baroque architecture, with its gaudily ornate designs, curved lines and ornamentation, had a stultifying influence on people and their thinking. Jenner was fortunate to have been born as it was coming to an end."

Not to be left out, and wishing to correct some of the preceding comments, Valerie Jones quickly interjected, "Don't forget good things also happened during the sixteenth and seventeenth centuries. Let's recall that the sixteenth century was outstanding for arts and letters, and more importantly, the seventeenth century has been labeled the 'golden age of science in Europe.' Others were even more generous and said it was the 'century of genius,' for it produced people like Newton, Galileo, Descartes, Pascal, Leibniz, Kepler, Boyle, Spinoza, Bacon, Huyghens, Locke and, oh yes, Harvey, the physician who discovered the circulation of the blood. Let's see that's twelve, but there are many more names that I could have added to the list."

Surprised and somewhat agitated by these comments, the Prof was quick to intervene. He wasn't going to permit anyone to go off on a tangent, and he attempted to get the conversation back to Jenner's boyhood. "Come, come, ladies, let's not judge the past too harshly. But I must say that was an impressive list of names that you mentioned, Valerie. I seriously doubt that I could come up with half that number on such short notice. Perhaps we can now, once again, focus our attention on Jenner. Valerie, please tell us something about Jenner's early development," knowing full well that she spent a great deal of her time, while in London, studying early English medical history.

To the Prof's dismay, before Valerie could continue, his wife, Iris, began speaking, "You know," she said, "Jenner lived during an important and exciting time in English history. Once England defeated the Spanish Armada in 1588, she developed a reputation as a world power and embarked on an extensive shipbuilding program that continued for centuries, so that, during the Jenner years, it was true, 'Britannia ruled the waves.'"

By now, the Prof was completely frustrated, but he knew better than to interrupt his wife, so he took the easy way out and said, "Yes. Go on, Iris. You were saying?"

"The English sea captains, Drake and Frobisher, never fully realized how those glorious ten days in July of 1588, changed our English nation, after they soundly defeated the Armada. By the time Jenner was born, England had somewhat over six million people, and London was the leading and most progressive city in Europe.

"About the time of Jenner's birth, another event was taking place that was changing how and where people worked. The industrial revolution was attracting workers, both men and women, to leave the farms for the big cities, where the factories and sweatshops were being built. In those industrialized cities, overcrowding and unsanitary living conditions prevailed, favoring the spread of infectious diseases, especially smallpox. During the eighteenth century, epidemics of smallpox and other infectious diseases caused so many deaths, among the skilled and unskilled working populations, that immigration was the only way the industrial revolution could continue to expand."

The Prof relaxed and relented, his voice no longer tentative, finally realizing that his wife was steering the conversation back to, and not away from Jenner. "Was there anything else you wanted to add?" he asked quietly.

"Well, yes," replied Iris, "It was Jenner's discovery that vaccination produced almost perfect immunity against smallpox which substantially reduced the death rate from the disease, and led directly to a dramatic increase in the world population. Without an increasing population to supply the needed manpower, the industrial revolution would have been impeded or completely stalled."

In order to reclaim the discussion, Valerie quickly commented, "Jenner was born in the western part of England in a parsonage, in the village of Berkeley, Gloucestershire, near the River Severn. It was, and still is, a small, country village, surrounded by streams and farms, and sheltered from the easterly winds that make their way across to the Severn River. The area was a wonderful place for a naturalist like Jenner to make discoveries about nature, and it was where he did his most significant work."

"The town of Berkeley was named for Berkeley Castle, which was built there," Murray Goldman was quick to point out. "The castle was famous—or infamous, whichever you prefer—as the place where King Edward II was murdered, in 1327."

"Thanks for your help, Murray," Valerie remarked sarcastically. She considered it rude for another person to interrupt when she was talking. It was somewhat out of character for Valerie to be so assertive. She enjoyed the lively discussions at Prof's house, and usually made her contributions in a soft voice and with an economy of words.

Valerie was a stunning brunet with her curly hair cut close to her nicely-shaped head. She had classical patrician features with lovely sparkling brown eyes. Her skin was a pale white which was a throwback to her Irish relatives. At age forty, she still maintained her slender figure, even after having had three children.

Valerie continued, "I should point out that the Berkeley family was very wealthy and influential in English politics. Edward's father had been the family's pastor and spiritual advisor. He tutored the children and was an intimate friend of the Baron. The close relationship of the two families would, one day, aid Edward in his fight to have vaccination accepted into English medicine." Valerie stopped for a moment, scanned the group for acceptance of what she was saying and carried on.

"Edward's father…"

◆   ◆   ◆

Edward's father was a vicar in the Church of England in the parish of Berkeley. He and his wife had six surviving children, of which Edward was the youngest. Unfortunately, both parents died suddenly, two months apart, in 1754, when Edward was five years old. It was an event that would indirectly change history, for instead of Edward going to Oxford and becoming a clergyman, as his father and brothers before him had done, he had to forego a classical theological education, due to the lack of finances, after his father died, and become a family doctor.

Starting at five years of age, a precocious Edward began to explore the Vale of Berkeley. Within the grassy meadows of the valley were the nests of many small creatures; along the shores of the Severn River were hidden the bones of large fish washed in from the sea; and entombed in the limestone cliffs bordering the valley were the skeletons of prehistoric animals. Even though exploring nature began at a young age, Jenner continued the practice for the remainder of his life. Solving nature's long held secrets that were concealed within and around the Vale of Berkeley would, one day, enable Edward to be elected into the Royal Society, England's most prestigious scientific club—but that was years away.

After his parents died, Stephen, his older brother, who had recently finished his theology studies at Oxford University, was assigned to a parish near Berkeley. Stephen elected not to marry. Instead he chose to care for Edward, acting as his surrogate father. It was a life-long responsibility that he honored until the day he died.

Edward was a well-disciplined child and accepted the religious beliefs that had been taught to him by his parents. Foremost he learned that while God may rule the universe, his parents ruled in the home.

After the parents died, Stephen explained to him that his parents were now happy with God, in Heaven. Due to his early religious training by his parents, before they died, Edward readily accepted this explanation, and expressed his feeling that, one day, he would like to join his parents in Heaven since "it must be such a happy place."

When Edward was about seven, he was sent off to school in the town of Wotton-under-Edge. For Edward, attending school with boys his own age was a happy experience, inasmuch as he easily made friends, and being a born naturalist, he was eager to show the boys how to explore the fields surrounding the school. Studying long hours was an essential part of the classical education that he was receiving. In spite of this, he was always able to find time to explore the fields and the meadows, searching out the nests of small rodents.

Unfortunately, for young Edward, eighteenth century England experienced a series of epidemics of smallpox, which brought calamities and catastrophes to a large part of the population, including the people of Wotton-on-Edge. The smallpox epidemic occurred when Edward was in school, and since Edward never had the disease, Stephen decided the safest thing for him was to be inoculated.

Since no one was expected to avoid the disease, most doctors used smallpox inoculation as the only means of prevention. Inoculation against smallpox continued even though serious illness—or sometimes death—could result from the procedure. The theory, established by Lady Montagu, was that it was wiser to undergo inoculation, hoping to get a mild form of the disease, rather than risk the more malignant form, when it was passed on naturally among susceptible individuals.

By the mid-eighteenth century, preparation for the inoculation had evolved into a formal ceremony so terrible that it was considered nearly as bad as having smallpox itself. Edward was subjected to six weeks of inhumane treatment, in preparation for the inoculation. First, he was put into isolation with other children that were also to be inoculated. The room where they were confined was dreary and frightening. Edward was given a starvation diet, followed by frequent bloodlettings, so his blood could be tested. Next, he was purged, over and over again, until he was puny and pathetic. During this time, he was forced to drink a vile concoction to "sweeten his blood." After completing his six weeks of torture, he was taken to a special stable. There he was harnessed with the other children, and they were all inoculated with an extract of smallpox material. Instead of a mild case of the disease, Edward developed a full-blown case of smallpox and came close to death. The originator of this brutal procedure was an apothecary who boasted, "But no one died."

For some time after the smallpox inoculation, Edward was depressed and melancholic. Parenthetically, melancholia was a sickness common in the eighteenth century. Throughout his life, Edward commented to his friends about his terrorizing experience, during his smallpox inoculation. These bitter memories were not wasted because, years later, the memory of them imbued Edward with the conviction that there had to be a better and more humane way of preventing smallpox.

After Edward recovered from the inoculation, Stephen had him transferred to a small school in Cirencester, which was under the charge of a famous tutor, a Rev. Dr. Washbourn. The school was closer to his home in Berkeley, and also nearer to the things of nature that he knew so well and with which he was comfortable. Edward was now in his element, and during this time, he gathered an enviable collection of dormice nests about which he lectured to anyone who would listen. Dr. Jenner was really a country boy at heart, and he would remain one all his adult life.

Whereas Edward's devotion to nature was foremost, the headmaster at the school, however, made sure that he received a classical education which included proficiency in the Latin language. Edward was taught grammar, not English grammar, but Latin grammar. The use of written Latin was still in fashion and supposedly was the preferred language of educated people. Greek grammar was also offered, but only to those boys going on to a university education.

It was about this time that Samuel Johnson published his monumental English dictionary which, one day, would enable English to become the common language of the country. Edward managed to get by in all his subjects but he did not excel in Latin grammar, while at school in Cirencester. Latin was a subject that he would struggle with all his life, and he was embarrassed, in later years, when attempting to translate letters, written in Latin, from his many friends abroad.

Observing nature was what Edward enjoyed the most. While he was at Cirencester, the nature studies of the renowned Swedish scientist, Linnaeus, were just being incorporated into the school's curriculum. Edward was pleased to learn that what he had considered to be his hobby was now a respected academic subject. It was at this school, at a young age, that he shaped friendships with a few of the boys that would last a lifetime.

By the age of twelve, Edward's grammar school days were over, and plans had to be made for his future. An academic career in either theology or medicine at Oxford University was not possible. Stephen had to sustain himself on a limited income from his parish, and lacked the funds to support Edward at Oxford. As an alternative, the family considered buying Edward a commission in the army or the navy, but even if they could have raised enough money, Edward wasn't suited for the life of an adventurer in the military; he enjoyed the country life too much, so the idea was discarded.

For Edward, careers suitable for a gentleman of his breeding were indeed limited. In the end, it was determined that he should study medicine and become a doctor—not at a university, but by serving an apprenticeship with a reputable country doctor.

In the eighteenth century, there were three ways to become a doctor: by qualifying at a university; serving an apprenticeship with a physician or a surgeon; or by being an apprentice to an apothecary. Edward was sent to study with an eminent surgeon, Mr. Daniel Ludlow, of Bristol. Mr. Ludlow had a busy medical and surgical practice and Edward would be taught the basic elements of medicine, surgery and pharmacy.

8

BY NOW THE LIVING ROOM WAS COLD, SO, ONE-by-one, the six people sitting on the couches got up, casually strolled to the huge fireplace and unabashedly presented their derrieres to the flames. They then began to vigorously rub their bottoms with both hands. It was an English custom that was acceptable in all the social classes. Of course, such an inelegant gesture was not needed by the Prof and Iris because, during the discussions, they were located close to the fireplace and its welcome warmth. Being strategically placed was carefully planned by them, after living in the old house for so many years, and they knew best how to survive in its challenging environment.

After the guests had sufficiently warmed themselves, they slowly ambled back to their places on the sofas, and the Prof immediately continued the discussion. "We know that Jenner completed his grammar school education at age twelve and, thereafter, he began his apprenticeship with the surgeon, Mr. Ludlow, at Sodbury.

"Iris, dear, please explain to our American friends why Ludlow was addressed as 'Mister' instead of 'Doctor,' even though his responsibilities were identical to those of many other physicians who were addressed as 'Doctor.' The division between the two terms is very English and isn't used in American medicine."

The Prof deliberately selected his wife, Iris, for the task since her father had been an eminent medical doctor and professor of medicine at Cambridge University. Iris, herself, was educated as a medical doctor, which few people realized. However, she never used the title "Doctor" on her stationery or when being introduced to company. In addition, as far as it is known, she never formally practiced medicine, even though she continually championed many worthy medical causes. All in all, Iris was an exceptional lady, more at home with the finer graces of the nineteenth rather than the twentieth century. Gentility and cultured tastefulness were conspicuous in her every movement. As a child she had a privileged upbringing. She never attended school until she entered the university; instead, Iris was tutored by a series of exceptionally fine private instructors, at home. All that is commendable in the French expression, *noblesse oblige*—rank imposes an obligation—she exemplified.

Iris always sat up straight in her chair, as if supported by a close-fitting undergarment, such as an old fashioned corset. Essentially, her posture was both charming and regal. When she was younger, Iris must have been an elegant young lady. She still had a fine, round face and laughing blue eyes. Her facial skin was unlined but slightly sallow. Iris was in her early sixties, a few years younger than her husband, and somewhat fleshy. She arranged everything in Prof's life, of which he was blissfully unaware: the house, the money, the children, the food, and his social calendar—all were carefully and discretely taken care of by Iris, over the years. Without her, the Prof would have been like a ship sailing aimlessly around in the ocean without a compass.

"If you will just give me a minute to step back in time, I'll oblige." Iris cleared her throat and began. "During the eighteenth century, there were many different types of people who cared for the sick, but most of them were charlatans or uneducated self-proclaimed doctors. The professional specialists that provided organized treatment for the sick were: first, the physicians, who were usually university educated and frequently were members of the Royal College of Medicine. They were the elite of the medical care system. Next, were the doctors, such as Jenner, who apprenticed themselves for many years to a qualified doctor or surgeon. The surgeons, early on, were known as barber-surgeons, functioning both as barbers and surgeons, in barbershops. By Jenner's time, many of the barber-surgeons were now capable surgeons and no longer acted as barbers. The apothecaries or pharmacists were supposed to only dispense medicines, but most of them didn't hesitate to also treat sick patients.

"Many of the early surgeons learned their trade in barber shops. In addition to being barbers, they did simple surgical procedures, sutured minor lacerations, extracted teeth, and so on; thus the generic term barber-surgeon was applied to them. Even during Jenner's time, there were still barber-surgeons of questionable character who were considered less than honest. These individuals tended to peddle their wares at fairs, where they attracted patients by salesmanship and false promises. Still, most were honest, conscientious, and dedicated to their patient's welfare. The skilled surgeons honed their surgical talents dissecting bodies of criminals that had been hanged, or bodies they bought from grave-robbers. The abilities and the reputation of the barber-surgeons improved markedly, from their origin in the middle-ages until the mid-fifteen hundreds, when they were organized and legitimized by being accepted into a Guild of Surgeons. The English surgeons elected to discard the title 'Doctor' and insisted on being called 'Mister.' It was the surgeon's way of reminding us of the time when every surgeon of distinction was a master surgeon of the Guild of Surgeons and carried the title 'Mister.'

Iris continued, "Mr. Ludlow..."

◆ ◆ ◆

Mr. Ludlow, to whom Jenner was apprenticed, was himself trained by a surgeon, thus his title "Mister." But his practice wasn't limited to surgery; he also cared for all kinds of medical aliments. More correctly, he was an old fashioned "country doctor." Edward's early training mainly involved helping Mr. Ludlow diagnose and treat his patients' illnesses. This assured Edward of an abundance of practical experience, but little in the way of theoretical knowledge, which could only be obtained from reading or lectures. Had he gone to medical school at either Cambridge or Oxford University, he would have had the opportunity to attend many medical lectures and complete numerous reading assignments; but he would have been exposed to little or no practical experience with patients.

Mr. Ludlow had a large country practice and kept Jenner busy as his assistant. A variety of illnesses were treated at the clinic, but surgical cases were frequent due to accidents and injuries, which were common in a farming community, where the roads were in poor repair. Travel by night was particularly dangerous and resulted in many injuries requiring surgery.

A considerable number of Mr. Ludlow's patients were local tradesmen, servants and farmers from the thriving market-town of Sodbury. But Mr. Ludlow's practice also extended well beyond the town, to encompass a vast farming community. Traveling on horseback enabled him to visit his patients in the rural areas. For the doctor, during those times, the horse was an essential part of his equipment.

Sodbury was a comfortable and convenient place for Edward to be. It was within riding distance from his home in Berkeley, and as he grew older, he frequently visited there and developed a close relationship with his brother Stephen, who had sacrificed much for him. But Sodbury also had other advantages, since it enabled Edward to continue with his nature studies. By now, these activities were an important part of Jenner's life.

Jenner was disappointed that he could not study medicine at a university, but that did not prevent him from engaging in his new medical studies with eagerness and enthusiasm. Mr. Ludlow was a demanding master and an excellent teacher, a combination of talents that enabled Edward to make rapid progress in his new profession. The Ludlows were an old and respected medical family in Sodbury, and they enjoyed having Edward living in their home. But above all, they respected him for his dedication and devotion to his medical work. In short order, his relationship with the family went beyond that of instructor and student; Edward was soon embraced as a family member.

During the eighteenth century, the practices of medicine and surgery were crude and, perhaps, even primitive in some ways. Nothing was known about germs and the diseases they caused. The "Germ Theory" was still a century away and needed scientists, such as Pasteur and Koch, to prove that microscopic organisms were the cause of many diseases.

Still, progress was being made. For example, advances in surgery were taking place at the great London hospitals, but, unfortunately, most of the surgery was performed by country doctors and continued to be somewhat primitive. Jenner spent much of his time as an apprentice, helping Mr. Ludlow saw off extremities, suture traumatic wounds and care for a variety of farming injuries. No matter how skilled the surgeon, the death rate after surgery was high, wounds frequently became infected and were a major cause of death. Unfortunately, for the patients, the cause of post-surgical wounds was unknown, since microorganisms had yet to be discovered. Rudimentary and crude ways of treating these infections were used, usually without success. Surgery was performed without an anesthetic. At times, large quantities of alcohol, in the form of gin or whiskey, were given to the patient, which was an ineffective way of controlling pain. During surgery, pain and suffering were common and a frequent cause of death.

The cause of fever was unknown, and, therefore, it was still being treated by bleeding the patient: by cupping or applying leeches. Sometimes, large amounts of blood were removed from a patient as a way of controlling the fever. Frequently, excessive blood was removed and caused the patient's death. Instruments used by the doctor for examining patients were limited. The stethoscope, for examination of the lungs and listening to the body sounds, had yet to be invented, and the thermometer was known but rarely used by the doctor. Neither the sterilization of surgical instruments nor hand-washing were thought to be necessary before or after surgery. Specialized obstetrical instruments had been devised for difficult deliveries; however, knowledge of their manner of use was limited to a small group of physicians. The use of medications by doctors was arbitrary; there were no fixed rules regarding how medicines were to be prescribed. Selection of a medicine was by choice, rather than specificity, and there were few medicines of any therapeutic value to the patient. Still, the plant containing digitalis was known to be a highly specific treatment for a person in heart failure, and sailors on long sea voyages, without any knowledge of ascorbic acid or vitamin C, ate fresh fruits or vegetables to prevent the disease, scurvy.

As an apprentice, Edward carefully cleaned the surgical instruments, washed the medicine bottles, dispensed the patients' medications and looked after the leeches used for bloodletting.

As Edward aged and gained in wisdom, his medical responsibilities increased. He ground and mixed his own herbs, as befitted the patient's illness, and rolled the pills and dispensed liquid medications of his own concoction. Later, he was permitted to bleed patients, which he did efficiently and with great care. Initially, during surgical procedures, his job was to prevent the patient from moving, but as he became more knowledgeable and efficient, he was permitted to saw off limbs and suture major lacerations, all under the watchful eye of Mr. Ludlow. Finally, Edward attained a degree of proficiency whereby he was permitted to care for the patient on his own. This was a major milestone for Edward, for he loved being a country doctor.

In a rural medical practice, the doctor had to journey long distances on coarse and choppy roads, which made traveling at night particularly dangerous. It became the custom for the doctor to stay the night in the farmer's home, and, if the situation warranted it, to remain for days.

Throughout the seven years of Edward's apprenticeship, smallpox ravaged a large area of England, including Sodbury and the surrounding towns, and while stopping over in a remote farming area, Edward was told of the farmers and dairymaids in the area who could not get smallpox infection. Later, while treating one of the dairymaids for another sickness, he was told the reason for her resistance to smallpox. The dairymaid casually remarked that she couldn't get the smallpox, because she already had had the cowpox. It was this chance remark, this unplanned utterance, which planted the seed in his mind that one day would lead to a discovery that would protect mankind from the terrible disease, smallpox. Only in the prepared mind will the seed of knowledge take root and grow, and Jenner's mind was prepared. Other doctors, before him, knew of the dairymaids who could not contract smallpox, because they previously had had cowpox, but they didn't have the vision or the ability of Jenner to carry this observation to its natural conclusion.

After seven years studying to be a doctor, Edward finally completed his apprenticeship, and it was time for him to leave Sodbury. In the interim, he changed from being a boy to that of a man. He was equally as efficient as his mentor, and was qualified to be a country doctor with his own practice. Fortunately for mankind, destiny intervened and changed the course of history. Stephen, Edward's brother and guardian, decided that he should continue his education in London, with Dr. John Hunter, one of the foremost doctors of his day and one of the great minds of the eighteen century.

9

"IN 1770, AT THE AGE OF 21, Jenner arrived in London and found Europe's most important city a densely populated metropolis," said the Prof. "Sarah what do you think?" Turning to the other guests, he smiled and said, "It is good to have an expert on London here with us tonight."

Sarah Foxworth was born in London and attended University College London where she majored in history and wrote her thesis on "The Eighteenth and Nineteenth Centuries London." She was a pretty English lady in her early forties, highly intelligent but inordinately shy and loath to speak out or to demonstrate her knowledge. Despite the fact that she wore eyeglasses, one immediately noticed her lovely, expressive, gray-blue eyes. She was slightly taller than the average female, perhaps five feet seven or eight, and thin to the extent of appearing anorexic. Her lovely auburn hair was drawn back and rolled into a chignon at the nape of her neck. Sarah was quieter than the rest of the people at the gathering and rarely initiated a conversation with the other guests. But hidden behind her painful timidity was an erudite English lady who, if she wished, could contribute much to the ongoing discussion, from her vast pool of knowledge.

"Well, perhaps. I'm sure, uh, uh. Don't you think someone else is more qualified to talk on this subject, uh, uh, than I am?"

"Nonsense." When he had to be, the Prof was an authoritarian figure even outside the laboratory, as on this occasion. "Come, come, let's get on with it, Sarah."

Forcefully, the Prof's wife, Iris, asserted her conjugal jurisdiction and came to Sarah's rescue. "Lawrence!" Everyone knew she was somewhat distressed when she addressed him as Lawrence, instead of the more homely term, Prof. "Please, Lawrence, give Sarah a chance to catch her breath. She needs time to think. You know Sarah will give us an excellent presentation, if you don't pressure her so."

Subjugated by a minimum of words, as can only be accomplished by one's mate, the Prof behaved contritely. "I'm sorry Sarah." No one believed that he really was sorry; he apologized only because he had been caught misbehaving. "Please, tell us about London, but only when you are ready."

Having been heartened by Iris's protective shield, Sarah responded. "I am hesitant to embark on describing London and its people during another century, a century that occurred so long ago. If we could visit eighteenth century London today, it would be as if we were visiting another country. The spoken and written languages were somewhat different from those presently in use. For example, reading a book would be difficult for some of us, since many of the printed words appear dissimilar, some of the letters bearing little resemblance to acceptable modern-day form.

"Besides, think how difficult it can be, in our own century, to completely understand each other, considering the many peculiarities in speech pronunciations and the variety of meanings that even a single word can convey. The meaning of a word can differ from country to country, as well as from generation to generation. For example, in America a lift is called an elevator; trousers are pants; a vest is an undershirt; knickers are called panties; petrol is gasoline—and so on.

"People are not only unique individuals within themselves, but they are also products of the area of the country in which they were born; the houses or buildings in which they grew up; the schools they attended; the stories they were told; the food they ate; and the faith they embraced. Anyway, I hope that you will overlook my limitations in attempting to describe for you what eighteenth century London and its people were really like. All that I can offer you is a narrow peek into the century from the vantage point of our own century, and hope that you will enjoy this brief intellectual jump back in time.

"By the mid-eighteenth century, London was a paradox. On the one hand, it was easily the most advanced city in Europe but, on the other hand, it was a hotbed of extreme poverty, licentiousness and disease, with smallpox the deadliest and most frightening disease of all.

"London, in…"

◆ ◆ ◆

London in 1770 was the right place to be for a young, intelligent doctor aspiring to advance in his profession. Over the course of 200 years, England had gradually developed into one of the most powerful countries in the world, with London as the center of English authority and prestige.

Eighteenth century London was the most impressive city in the west, with its many churches dominating the skyline. The population of over one-half million people comprised one-tenth of the entire English population. With a multitude of boats traversing its waters daily, the river Thames was one of the main channels of communication, commerce and travel. Small shops and houses lined London Bridge, which was the only bridge connecting the north and south shores. Down from the bridge was the Port of London, where ships from around the world unloaded their valuable cargoes. It was this wealth that sustained the vigorous economy of the city. However, the city couldn't continue to grow without immigration, since deaths outnumbered births, with smallpox being the major contributor to its high death rate.

No one was exempt from smallpox: neither the rich nor poor; commoner nor royalty; young nor old. Not only English royalty, but all the royal houses of Europe felt the sting of this vicious disease. At the time of Elizabeth I, who suffered through two attacks of smallpox, England became a world-class naval power, able to defeat the pride of Spain, the formidable Spanish Armada. During Elizabeth's reign, the first English New World colonies were established. Trade with these colonies and the rest of the world was what made England rich and powerful; and it was the English Navy and Merchant Marine that enabled her to engage in such a robust and productive international trade. Along with the latter, came the wealth that supported the growth and development of her cities, particularly London.

With wealth came power, and with power came the drive for exploration and annexation. Sir Robert Clive, previously a clerk in the East India Company, used his military genius to establish the British Empire in India; and Captain Cook laid claim to Australia and New Zealand for the Crown, during his daring sea voyages of exploration.

With military brilliance came pomp and ceremony, an important part of the social life of London. The distinguished Admiral Lord Horatio Nelson was acclaimed for his victory over the French fleet at Trafalgar, off the coast of Spain, while the Duke of Wellington was much honored for his victory over the indefatigable Napoleon at Waterloo, in Belgium. Both these remarkable generals, Wellington and Napoleon, knew of Jenner's discovery for the prevention of smallpox by the use of vaccination, and they were among the first to have their soldiers vaccinated. It wasn't long before the English navy, too, vaccinated all its sailors. Wellington and Napoleon held Jenner in the highest esteem. They were proud, arrogant and haughty generals, regarding their reputations as military geniuses, but they also knew that defeat on the battlefield was inevitable, if their armies were weakened or destroyed by smallpox, the most feared of all their enemies.

For Jenner, London was a physical marvel to behold, since it had been newly rebuilt, after it was destroyed by the Great Fire of 1666. The fire provided a sorely overdue catharsis or cleansing of the city, a much needed renewal, similar to a forest fire that burns away the dead, rotting trees and underbrush and makes way for an abundance of new life. So, too, the Great Fire eliminated the old rot, filth and germs of London, enabling the city to have a fresh beginning.

Jenner witnessed the best and the worst of London and its environs, as he traveled to the home of Dr. John Hunter, with whom he would live and study for the next two years. Suddenly, as Jenner's carriage approached the city, he was overcome by a horrible stench, forcing him to cover his nose with his handkerchief. He looked out the carriage window and saw the cause of his discomfort. The area was rife with piles of garbage, discarded there by the homeless "night people" that wandered about the city. The city streets and trenches were filled with human bodily waste and urine, while the mud-covered roadways were a potent mixture of horse droppings, along with other animal excrements. As the carriage passed by London's jam-packed cemeteries and charnel houses, the odor of unburied bodies added to the unbelievably offensive smells of the city.

Still, as Jenner's carriage penetrated deeper into London, he was overcome with emotion upon seeing the magnificence and richness of the city. Much of the splendor of the city was the work of one man who epitomized discerning reason, discriminating wit and discreet genius—the architect and builder, Sir Christopher Wren. The biographer, James Boswell, in 1763, climbed to the dome of St. Paul's cathedral, one of Wren's magnificent creations, in an attempt to take in all of London in one spectacular panoramic view. His daring deed was without satisfaction though, as he remarked after he descended, "All I saw were the tiled roofs and narrow lanes opening here and there." But the view of London, for Jenner, was very different at ground level from his carriage window. Even though it was early morning when he entered the city, there were people in motion everywhere, mainly servants gathering coal to light fires in the bedrooms, kitchens and dining rooms of the stylish London homes. But from the chimneys of these same homes, ugly clouds of black smoke belched forth and covered the streets, like a black drape covering a bier. For a young man nurtured on the sweet pure country air of Berkeley, the pollutants, discharged into the air by the burning of the deadly bituminous coal in the fireplaces of London, were overwhelming. His carriage passed through sections of the city where the inhalation of the carbon particles made it almost impossible for him to breathe. He was again forced to cover his nose and mouth with his handkerchief, which was quickly turned black by the microscopic carbon particles that clung to it. At that moment, Jenner's focus of attention was his lungs, which he visualized changing from their normally soft pink color to that of a rigid and perverse black.

Still, it was the beauty of Wren's architectural genius, with his spires, steeples and Roman Doric columns, that inspired him, and Jenner was infatuated with the aesthetic richness of Wren's work. However, there was also the London that Samuel Johnson, the great lexicographer, knew and wrote about. It was this depressing aspect of London that stirred the young Jenner's humane nature. Large sections of the city were appalling. Deaths outnumbered births by a ratio of two to one, with the ubiquitous and murderous smallpox always present, and a major cause of death. There was a constant cacophony of bells pealing, to signify when a person died. The sonorous tolling of the bells seemed to be constant, and this background noise was heard throughout the city.

Actually, the city was alive with many different sounds, which one could differentiate by listening carefully: merchant peddlers extolling their goods; chimney sweeps hawking their services; itinerant craftsmen offering to mend shoes or sharpen knives; putrid and polluted prostitutes wailing their willingness to perform their services for a few pence. These were the common sounds of the city, along with the shrieks, moans and incoherent babble of drunkenness and debauchery; for gin was cheap and one of the favored intoxicants of the poorer classes. The cobblestones lining the streets also contributed to the discordant sounds of the city, as Jenner's carriage wheels passed over them. How different from the tranquil village of Berkeley, where he could savor the soft sound of the exhilarating breeze as it brushed gently past his ears.

Death and disease were constant companions of all Londoners. An epidemic of smallpox could kill all the children in a family within days. Thousands of young children failed to reach adulthood, for children were the most susceptible. The killer smallpox was so contagious and frightening that there were times when the clergy refused to bury the dead. London was so riddled with diseases, that a third of its population failed to reach the age of fifty. Funerals were a common sight, and the services of undertakers and coffin-makers were in constant demand. The death rate in London, during the time Jenner was there, was the highest that it had been during the previous century, and without the constant influx of new blood, the city would have been badly depleted of its source of energy—its working population. Attempts were made at recording the causes of death in a 'Bill of Mortality,' which was the start of public health record-keeping. While such records were extensive, they were also unreliable, since a certificate of death from a doctor was not required. The cause of death was usually based upon hearsay or a cursory examination by an inexperienced, elderly neighborhood lady. The infectious diseases, plague and smallpox, however, were exceptions, as they were the only two that could be easily and accurately identified by either doctor or layman.

For the past two hundred years, the practice of medicine was under the jurisdiction of the College of Physicians of London. By examinations and licensing, the College controlled who was qualified to practice medicine, and, in this way, they had hoped to prevent charlatans, quacks and the apothecaries from illegally treating patients. Most troublesome were the apothecaries; while they were, theoretically, limited to only dispensing drugs, they actually treated a large share of London's sick.

But the system of medical care in London was archaic, unacceptable and inadequate. A half-million Londoners were supposed to receive their medical care from sixty to eighty physicians who belonged to the College of Physicians. The College argued that, to care for patients and prescribe medicines, practitioners were required to be knowledgeable in both Latin and Greek; and the true physicians were only those individuals who had spent fourteen years studying medicine at either Oxford or Cambridge University. Unfortunately though, a university medical education was based upon the archaic teachings of Hippocrates, born in 460 B.C., and Galen, born in 130 A.D.

As is frequently the case, the medical wisdom of the times is pitilessly expressed in its wit: "Wise men were advised to avoid the greedy physicians who had a vested interest in over-prescribing worthless medicines. But when a sick man leaves all to nature, he also risks much. On the other hand, to leave all to the physician, he risks even more. Considering that there are risks both ways, it was better to trust nature, for we can be sure that nature acts honestly and does not become richer by prolonging the disease."

In fact, all types of tradesmen, charlatans and quacks treated the sick, especially the poor. Few, if any, medicines were of any value and most herbs and herbal concoctions were equally worthless, except, perhaps, the flowers of the purple foxglove plant which contained the heart stimulant, digitalis.

Bloodletting was still used as a treatment for most ailments, and people admitted to having it performed on a yearly basis, as a way of purifying their blood, which was thought to accumulate toxic substances.

The barber-surgeons, the forebears of modern surgery, were similarly maligned by The College of Physicians, even though many had a more detailed practical knowledge of the human body than did the physicians. To be recognized as a surgeon required a seven-year apprenticeship and membership in the Worshipful Company of Barber-Surgeons. While the barbers and surgeons usually were members of the same organization, they were restricted to the practice of their own particular specialty.

By virtue of the fact that injuries and accidents were commonplace in the congested streets of London, the services of the surgeons were in constant demand. Some form of alcohol was used to quiet the patient during surgery, but alcohol was of little value in preventing severe pain and, therefore, speed and dexterity were the surgeon's greatest assets. Knowledge of sterilization was still a century away; accordingly, the surgeons' dirty hands and instruments infected and killed as many patients as were saved.

Surgery was mainly limited to the removal of external organs, such as broken limbs, mastectomies and external tumors. Suturing lacerations, resulting from accidents and knife wounds, kept the surgeons busy. Operations inside the body were uncommon; however, cutting into the abdomen for renal stones did take place, but the outcome was frequently the death of the patient. It seems that as many patients died of the operations as died of the stones.

Cannabis—marijuana—available in the apothecary shops, was used for coughs, asthma and a host of other diseases. Opium too could be obtained from the chemist but its toxic effects were poorly understood, so that most people avoided using it.

The doctrine of Galenic medicine, dating back sixteen-hundred years, still pervaded eighteenth century English medicine. Galen held that the cause of disease was an imbalance in the four body humours: blood, phlegm, yellow and black bile; and to restore the balance of the humours, the treatments of choice were bloodletting, cupping and the use of leeches.

But, still, medical theories based upon scientific research were slowly evolving, under the leadership of the doctors at the free hospitals for the poor and aged of London. In the sixteenth century, with the closing of the monasteries, hospitals such as St. Bartholomew and St. Thomas came into existence, utilizing their abandoned buildings. In these hospitals, or confiscated monasteries, a humble form of nursing had its beginnings. The nurses were called "Sisters," a salutation carried over from the nuns who previously had occupied the monasteries. Bethlehem Hospital, known as Bedlam, previously a monastery, was the only public asylum for the insane, and thus the word, "bedlam" has become associated with the concept of insanity.

Spas seem to have developed out of a need for some form of treatment for the common chronic diseases. The London drinking water was contaminated, so the use of fresh drinking and bathing water at the spas was conceived as a healthful means of treating disease. Unfortunately, this form of treatment was frequently restricted to the more affluent members of society. The earliest spa in England was established by the Romans in the city of Bath, and at a later date, an equally famous spa was established in the town of Cheltenham. It was the people of Cheltenham who were the early supporters of Jenner and his use of vaccination in the fight against smallpox; and it was where he lived and practiced medicine in the latter part of his life.

The Cheltenham spa was begun, when pigeons were seen pecking at the salt deposits at the periphery of the springs. Their action was interpreted as being symbolic with health, and shortly thereafter, the spring water was promoted as a 'cure-all' for practically all chronic diseases. However, it wasn't until King George III visited Cheltenham for treatment that the medicinal value of the spa's water was accepted.

Eighteenth century society was still divided into strictly defined classes, and clothing was one way of proclaiming where a person stood in the hierarchy of the social system. Royalty had its own special apparel symbols of rank. For wealthy Londoners, the wearing of expensive clothes on special occasions, such as, attendance at church, the opera or societal parties, was their way of gaining esteem. A well-dressed female was an asset to her family or her husband, but an overly-dressed male was known as a fop and was subjected to ridicule or humor. In dress, the working-class tended to mimic the upper social class, and well designed second-hand clothing was readily available to them. For the poor, clothing was nothing more than a means for keeping warm in the winter and dry when it rained.

A man was born a gentleman by ancestral right, and without that fortunate accident of birth, no amount of good breeding or financial gain could change his status; thus there was a wide gap between gentlemen and the other classes of society. A gentleman-by-birth was assured special treatment by those less fortunate, but the *nouveau riche*, who lacked a superior line of ancestors, was frequently taunted, especially by the novelists of the period.

The merchants comprised another distinct social group. The accumulation of large fortunes in business was common, and the moneyed class had so much political influence, that the old stigma of trade was now beginning to disappear. It was observed by a foreigner that "in England, commerce is not looked down upon as being disdainful, as it is in France and Germany. Here men of good family, and even rank, may become merchants, without losing caste (social status)."

Jenner, as he entered London to study with John Hunter, was among a group of young progressive doctors who were about to change the face of medicine, and he, one day, would be recognized for the leadership role that he played in helping to establish the scientific age of medicine in England.

10

WHEN THE WOMEN BEGAN TO SQUIRM, the Prof finally noticed that he had neglected the fire, and the room had become quite chilly. His female guests were beginning to react noticeably to the drop in temperature.

"Lawrence, do something to the fire; can't you see the ladies are cold?" questioned Iris.

For the Prof, the question was an extraneous one, for he could neither see cold nor determine the body temperature of other people by looking at them. In fact, a person's state of being would, most likely, go unnoticed by the Prof, since there was no way for him to calculate it mathematically or to apply some bizarre analytical formula to reach an answer.

"Noise! Yes," he thought. It was the noise, of course; the fact that the women began making discernible little sounds, as they wiggled in their seats, that made him aware the fire had died down.

Suddenly, Iris gave her most direct command, "Lawrence!" The name was said with some force, as if to bring him out of a trance. "Please, put some logs on the fire and stir it up, because we are all chilly." It was as if she could read his mind; she knew that he was fantasizing with words and ideas and not getting on with solving the problem of the waning flames.

Once the Prof was properly instructed by his wife, he immediately directed his attention to the fire. Three thick logs, cut to size, were nearby and, in turn, were placed on top of the smoldering remains of the fire. There is some sort of close relationship between a log fire and the person attending it that is not readily explainable. For example, each person seems to have his own unique method of using the poker to stir up a fire, so that it will give the maximum amount of heat in the shortest length of time. And the Prof was no exception to the rules of conduct governing the care of a log fire, for he poked and moved the logs in his own special way, as though the ritual could not be performed properly by anyone else in the room.

While all this was going on, the women began exchanging glances and whispering to one another, their comments evoking muffled giggles amongst themselves. By this time, the liquid they had ingested at dinner and afterwards had filtered its way down to their bladders, which were now pleading for relief. Moreover, the chilly room itself added additional impulses to their bladders' increasing feelings of urgency. The question the ladies were quietly addressing was which one of them would be the bravest to venture to the water closet, or privy, where the temperature was equal to or lower than the outside temperature. Besides, the frigid privy seat always seemed to be the coldest object in the house. How the ladies determined who would be the first to make a move is unknown but, one by one, they marched down the cold hallway. By the time this ceremony was concluded, the Prof had the log fire blazing, and the room was once again becoming more comfortable.

"Well, Cedric?" the Prof wished to begin a new conversation and addressed his remarks to Cedric Foxworth, who was familiar with the historical developments of English medicine. "We now have Dr. Jenner going to London, to advance his career by studying with a Dr. John Hunter. Why Hunter?"

Cedric was never at a loss for words and enjoyed dominating a conversation. "Before we get on to Dr. Hunter, Prof, I would like to say something about how English medical doctors learned their anatomy. The dissection of corpses was essential to the teaching of anatomy and surgery. Up until the middle of the eighteenth century in England, after being hanged at the gallows, the bodies of criminals were given to doctors to be dissected for the study of anatomy. At the time, the dissection of corpses was laden with religious deliberations and taboos. For example, popular sentiment held that dismemberment of criminals, after hanging, prevented them from ever resting in peace or attaining heaven. Nevertheless, the demand for bodies for dissection was so great that soon the bodies of all criminals who died in prison were relinquished for teaching purposes.

"Then, in 1752, a law was passed limiting the number of bodies of criminals allotted to any one doctor for anatomical dissection or surgical demonstrations. While the law meant well, restricting the number of criminal corpses deprived doctors of the bodies they needed for demonstration purposes, and from keeping abreast of the medical and surgical advancements taking place. Ultimately, to compensate for this critical shortage, a new, laborious and dangerous enterprise evolved, to meet the doctors' needs. Shady, disreputable characters known as body-snatchers or grave-robbers, now filled the gap, by supplying the badly needed bodies. Though it was an immoral and dishonest business, still, it persisted through the remainder of the century. Choice London cemeteries were continually violated. In the end, body-snatching was so common that, at night, guards and mastiff dogs were needed to patrol the graveyards; regardless, by morning, both the corpses and the dogs would be missing.

"When Dr. Jenner finished his apprenticeship with Mr. Daniel Ludlow, the surgeon in Sodbury, he had hoped to begin his own medical and surgical practice in Berkeley, his hometown. Concerned that Edward had been deprived of a university medical degree, Stephen, now a parish rector with an adequate income, decided to enable him to advance his medical and surgical knowledge by arranging for him to complete his studies in London with one of the foremost surgeons, scientists and teachers of the eighteenth century, John Hunter.

"At the time when Edward was first eligible to attend University, to attain a medical degree, Stephen lacked the finances to support him. The absence of a proper university medical degree vexed Dr. Jenner the better part of his medical career, even though, in 1792, St. Andrew's College, Scotland, awarded him the degree of Doctor of Medicine.

"There are events in everyone's life that are pivotal, and for Dr. Jenner it was when he went to London to study with Dr. John Hunter. Was it luck, fate, or something else that directed Jenner to study with Hunter? Perhaps, it was all these things combined. Still, any one explanation may be true—or false—who knows? Conceivably though, the old adage that best applies to Dr. Jenner's joining Hunter is: 'Your destiny will find you.'

"No description of…"

◆   ◆   ◆

No description of eighteenth century medicine would be complete without alluding to the brothers, William and John Hunter. William, the older brother, left Scotland first, in order to advance his career in London. When he arrived there, he was fortunate to have been invited to study with one of the foremost London anatomists. After his patron died, he established the Windmill Street School of Anatomy which, for years, was the leading center of anatomical instruction in London. William, a courtly and elegantly dressed man, soon became the leading obstetrician in London and was invited to become the obstetrician for the women of the royal family, an honor which brought him both fame and fortune. Foremost among his many successful endeavors were his female anatomical and obstetrical drawings, which were so anatomically accurate and life-like that they were used for teaching purposes for the next two centuries.

Despite his intellectual and medical abilities, his younger brother, John Hunter, would, one day, surpass him in intellectual and academic achievements, although William surpassed John in the social graces. However, John was the youngest of eleven children and, from the beginning, he was driven to excel. It was a trait that would remain with him until the day he died.

John Hunter was eventually invited by William to join him at his London anatomical school. John did, and he quickly became an excellent anatomist. A short time later, he was invited to study surgery with two of the leading surgeons in London. It wasn't long before John established himself as a talented surgeon and a distinguished comparative anatomist, a subject for which he was soon to become world famous.

Surgery, before long, became just a means by which John could support his research in comparative anatomy. Eventually, his comparative anatomy collection numbered nearly fourteen thousand specimens, which became the basis of his world renowned museum.

After leaving William's anatomical and surgical school on Windmill Street, John decided to establish his own school for training in surgery and comparative anatomy. Jenner, at the age of 21 years, was Dr. Hunter's first pupil. The two doctors immediately took a liking to each other, even though Hunter was 20 years older than his pupil.

When Jenner arrived at Hunter's house on Jermyn Street in London, it served as his home, school and research laboratory. It was essentially a bachelor household, since neither Hunter nor Jenner was married. Both men followed a rather rigidly precise routine, which began early each morning. Unlike most men of their class, who remained in bed in the morning and drank their hot chocolate, and then spent a good part of the morning dressing, Hunter and Jenner, by six in the morning, were in the dissecting room ready to start a long day of work.

During the two years that Jenner lived and studied with Hunter, they learned to respect each other's abilities, even though they had quite different personalities. Hunter tended to be short-tempered, gruff and abrasive, and was noted for his rages and bouts of swearing; while Jenner was the opposite: quiet, retiring and gentle, though still highly intelligent. The two remained close friends and associates, until Hunter died in 1793.

The two men contrasted in appearance as well as temperament. Jenner was stocky, of medium height, with a round face and a pale complexion. His eyes were bright and the focus of attention; lips were well formed and full; chin was strongly structured, suggesting determination and strength of character; hair was light and neatly combed in a club, or roll, in the back. He dressed tidily, as a gentleman, though not that of an English dandy. Hunter, on the other hand, was thinner and slightly shorter in stature than his student. His piercing eyes and thin lips suggested a firm directness of manner. His dress was casual and unpretentious, and he loathed to change his suit, which was usually stained with blood and exudates from the cadavers on which he had been working.

After Jenner had spent seven years studying conservative, old-fashioned medicine with Mr. Ludlow, he was knowledgeable in the standard treatment for nearly all the known diseases. When his treatment failed, he was told that the fault was never in the remedy, but in the patient, the disease, or some anomaly in the patient's makeup. Hunter, on the other hand, introduced Jenner to a new way of thinking; if his treatment failed, it was because it was the wrong treatment. "Take nothing for granted. Think, plan and experiment," Hunter repeated over and over again. Hunter demanded the facts, which had to be checked by experimenting. Jenner found it all new, exciting and intellectually stimulating.

After working all morning in the laboratory, precisely at the stroke of noon, Hunter left for his surgical rounds, with Jenner following close behind. No one knew better than Hunter the crudeness of the surgery that was being practiced, and he was determined to change surgery from a form of carnage into an acceptable science. No matter how much money he earned from his surgery, it all went to support his research and comparative anatomy museum. Hunter set a good example for Jenner, who quickly learned that he would have to search out new knowledge; it was not adequate merely to "become a doctor."

Fortunately, the training Jenner received, under Hunter's tutelage would prove to be of inestimable value to him, on his path to becoming an outstanding physician and researcher. Jenner easily followed Hunter's rigid patterns of punctuality, because they coincided, more or less, with his own good habits. Exactly at two o'clock in the afternoon, Jenner completed his hospital duties with Hunter, and then proceeded to his place in the anatomy lecture theater. The anatomy lectures were extremely popular and not necessarily the exclusive prerogative of the medical students and the doctors; equal numbers of art students from the Royal Academy also attended.

In the evenings, Jenner could be found back in the laboratory dissecting his specimens and mounting them for the museum. Hunter never forced Jenner to use the medical literature, which he claimed was meager to begin with and, in general, unscientific. Instead, he insisted that medical knowledge must be obtained by research in the dissecting room.

On occasion, Jenner's curiosity moved him to explore the back streets of London. At times, he walked across St. James' Park and on into the Mall, a fashionable place to walk in the daytime. In the evening, however, it was an area of dubious reputation, and it was here that the great Boswell met his lewd lovers, and thievery was practiced with impunity in the shadowy darkness. One day, Jenner walked past Hyde Park to an area that on that day of the week, a Monday, was the scene of hangings. Thousands of people gathered to take part in the holiday spirit associated with the executions. Stalls which sold cakes and sweetmeats were everywhere. Music, the singing of ballads, and recitation of poetry proclaiming that crime does not pay, filled the air. Undoubtedly, the poor, wretched souls awaiting the hangman were thoroughly confused by the goings-on.

Since it was a Christian society, the prisoners were accompanied by a chaplain, in the cart taking them to the gallows. The chaplain tried to convince the men—it was usually men—that they were "on their way to heaven," as if the prisoners weren't aware of it, seeing their coffins were being carried close behind the cart. Friends were on hand to offer them their condolences, and pull on their legs as they were hanged, to shorten their period of dying. After the hanging, it was their friends who fought off the body-snatchers, in order to obtain the bodies for decent burials. It was a brutal day's outing for the gentle natured Jenner; a scene he most likely would have preferred not to witness. Jenner quickly left the area and moved on to explore what he hoped would be more agreeable sections of London. In general, Jenner was never comfortable in London and he often admitted to his friends that he developed a strong, permanent dislike for the city.

Hunter's home was a beehive of intellectual and cultural activity, and the gathering place for many distinguished individuals. In 1771, Sir Joseph Banks, a naturalist, recently returned from his round-the-world voyage with Captain Cook, met Jenner at Hunter's home. Banks was so impressed with Jenner's work, and knowledge of animals and plants, that he offered him the place as naturalist on Captain Cook's up-and-coming second round-the-world expedition. Jenner politely declined, for he was anxious to continue his own work and return to Berkeley as a country doctor. Banks eventually became president of the Royal Society, England's most prestigious scientific society, and one day he would welcome Jenner into the Society and acknowledge him for his scientific achievements.

Science was only part of Jenner's life in London, for Hunter eventually married and brought home a highly cultured and talented wife, who was a celebrity in her own right, the Scottish poetess, Anne Home. Anne was also interested in painting, amongst her numerous talents, and had accumulated an imposing art collection. It was Anne who introduced the shy and reserved Jenner to the world of art. Under Anne's guidance, Jenner became knowledgeable in art, as well in literature; and he became interested in music, to the extent that he took up playing the violin and the flute. The great composer, Haydn, was a friend of Anne's and a frequent visitor to the Hunter home, and hence became a friend of Jenner. In addition to her other talents, Anne Hunter was a composer and lyricist, and had contributed lyrics for some of Haydn's compositions.

At the time Jenner arrived in London, economic and sociologic changes were taking place throughout England. These rudimentary changes would later become known in the western world as the Industrial Revolution. It was the replacement of hand tools with machines and power tools, and the movement of people from the small towns to the large cities, that stimulated and propelled the revolution. Changes had been occurring slowly over decades, and as the revolution grew, London became the financial center which fed the flames of expansion.

During the last half of the eighteenth century, London had witnessed unprecedented growth, not only in population and wealth, but in culture as well. The stylish notion of high culture is an artifice of eighteenth century London. Explosive growth occurred in art, literature and the theater. At the same time, new cultural associations came into being, and philosophical questions were argued about the relationship between art and society.

It was this new London scene to which the young Jenner was exposed; however, because of his small, country-town rearing, he was never quite able or willing to adjust to the extremes of the London environment.

Besides London being a financial center, it needed population growth to sustain an ever increasing industrial growth that one day would be classified as a revolution. However, the limiting factor on the growth of the population was disease, and smallpox was the leading killer and destroyer, particularly of the younger population, in the leading industrial cities of England. Some have speculated that, without Dr. Jenner's cowpox vaccination and control of the cruel smallpox, the industrial revolution in England would have been markedly delayed.

To understand John Hunter's great influence on Jenner, it is imperative to comprehend Hunter and his extraordinary rise to success in the world of medicine and science. When John Hunter rode into London, in 1750, he was a twenty-one year-old good-for-nothing, idler, layabout and trifler, and within 20 years, by the time Jenner went to study with him, in 1770, he was a renowned surgeon and anatomist, and had established the world's leading comparative anatomy museum in his home.

While growing up, John Hunter, born in 1728, rejected the limits placed upon him in the process of obtaining a formal education. He wanted to know much more than he was being taught. John was terribly bright, and this unruly boy wished to know about the things of nature and how they worked: why the leaves turned color; what the clouds were made of; and he observed in detail the behavior of the bees, birds, ants, tadpoles and worms. He asked questions that other people weren't interested in or were unable to answer.

When he arrived at his brother, William's, anatomy laboratory on Windmill Street in London, John was assigned menial jobs, commensurate with his lack of a formal education. He lived and slept at the laboratory, where he received the corpses that were delivered surreptitiously in the middle of the night, by shabby individuals of disreputable character. With these unsavory individuals, he was famous for haggling and dickering, and within the community of body-snatchers, he was known to drive a "Scotsman's bargain," with no questions asked. He lived and slept with the dead felons and eventually dissected their diseased bodies. While his living and working conditions were disgusting and loathsome, with odors that were nauseating, John never once complained. In fact, he worked beyond the limits of an ordinary man, so much so, that his brother feared he would have a break-down and his health would become impaired.

During the daytime, John accompanied William to the hospital, to assist in surgery and caring for the patients. His nights were spent dissecting and mounting various parts of the human body. While dissecting was tedious and detailed, he excelled at it, and seemed to be oblivious to his noxious surroundings. Eventually, John displayed such a gift for his work that, in 1753, William offered to make him a partner.

In due time, John qualified as an apprentice surgeon, but as William feared, John's health began to deteriorate, due to the intensity of his grueling work habits. To enable his brother to recover his health, William obtained for him an appointment as surgeon at a military hospital.

It was a posting that William thought would be less strenuous and demanding, but what William failed to realize was that John would apply the same intensity to his new assignment as he did to his work in the past.

Since the Seven Years War was going on, John was sent as a military surgeon to the battle at Belle Isle. It was a place where the surgeons were overwhelmed with hundreds and hundreds of casualties. As usual, Hunter showed his independent spirit and began treating the wounded with new and innovative techniques of his own creation. By disregarding accepted military surgical procedures, he made himself many enemies. His scathing, sarcastic remarks about the obsolescent procedures being followed by his fellow surgeons were not kindly received. Hunter was never hesitant to denounce what he considered poor or improper treatment of medical or surgical patients. From his military experiences, caring for the wounded, he published his excellent treatise on the proper care and treatment of gunshot wounds.

After the war, in 1763, he returned to London and began practicing medicine as a surgeon. However, his lack of formal university medical training was a problem in upscale London. Fortunately, however, his experience and training as a military surgeon soon enabled him to establish a sterling reputation for himself.

Because John lacked the graces of an educated man, William decided to send him to Oxford University, hoping to make him a scholar and a gentleman, but this venture failed. After attending an Oxford medical lecture, John was known to remark that he found the Oxford lecture more nauseating and less informative than living and working with the decaying corpses the body-snatchers brought to him. It was not a flattering remark about a university medical education but, probably, was close to the truth for the times. With that, John left Oxford for good, and returned to London where he became one of the pioneers in modern, scientific medicine and surgery.

At his own school, Hunter became famous for his lectures on surgery as well as comparative anatomy—the study of human and animal structures, organs and parts which are similar in function. His work in Comparative Anatomy and preservation of human and animal tissues led to many honors, and eventually, to his being elected as a Fellow of the Royal Society, the most prestigious scientific appointment, at that time.

As a pupil of John Hunter, Jenner found that his work was hard and the hours were long. During the day, Jenner worked with Hunter at St. George's Hospital taking care of patients and assisting him in surgery. Besides these duties, there were many small chores which he had to perform, and he was also expected to attend lectures in anatomy, pathology, pharmacy and midwifery. However, the day didn't end there since, in the evening, Jenner was required to carry on with his own research and to assist Hunter with his.

The long hours and demanding work meant nothing to either man, since their main desire was the proper care of their patients, and after that to advance medical knowledge for the good of all mankind. Neither doctor used his medical knowledge for the primary purpose of enriching himself financially, and they both respected and lived by the Hippocratic Oath that they swore to, when they became physicians. Hippocrates, the Greek physician who lived over two thousand years ago, established an oath which all physicians were—and are—expected to follow. In part it reads: "I will prescribe regimen for the good of my patients, according to my ability and my judgment, and never do harm to anyone."

In the intense two years together, an extraordinary comradeship and empathy was established between the two doctors, and for the remainder of his life, Jenner would refer to John Hunter as, "the dear man." Jenner not only respected his teacher, but he loved the man. The doctors shared a directness and plainness of conduct, and their insatiable craving for knowledge, along with an inextinguishable love of truth. In reality, the two years in London that Jenner spent working with Hunter were more valuable to him than any university education would have been.

After Jenner left London, the two men frequently wrote to each other and exchanged scientific information. Hunter continued to request samples of animals and plants that were only available in the Berkeley area and along the Severn River.

Before long, Hunter sorely missed Jenner and offered him an opportunity to become his partner in surgery, research and teaching in the London Hospitals, but Jenner refused, wishing to remain as a family doctor in the countryside of Berkeley, an area that he dearly loved.

At times, life takes an unusual turn. During the years that Jenner was in practice in Berkeley, he was the first physician to report that the chest pain, which is later associated with heart failure and death, is due to degenerative changes in the coronary arteries of the heart. While dissecting the body of a man who died after strenuous physical work and who previously had had severe chest pain, he observed abnormal coronary arteries. This unusual type of chest pain was named angina pectoris by another physician, a Dr. Heberden. Jenner had written to Heberden about his discovery that angina pectoris was due to a blockage of the coronary arteries. Jenner's humanism is obvious in his letter to Heberden: "How much the heart must suffer from the coronary arteries not being able to perform their function."

It was in 1777 that Jenner learned that his friend, "the dear man," Dr. Hunter, was suffering from chest pain, angina pectoris. Hunter knew nothing of Jenner's discovery, and Jenner was reluctant to tell him what was causing his pain, since he could offer no treatment. Jenner feared that if Hunter knew of his finding, he would be deprived of all hope of recovery. Unfortunately, Jenner's diagnosis of Hunter's chest pain was correct. Hunter died of coronary disease, in 1793, following a strenuous argument with a colleague.

Hunter was the near-perfect physician, because the care of his patients was foremost; he studied and kept up-to-date with the latest in medical knowledge, so that his patients would benefit; he did basic research for a greater understanding of disease, so, in the long run, all humanity would benefit; and he handed down the torch of knowledge to those doctors who would follow him. In the end, Hunter directly or indirectly handed the torch to thousands of doctors, but the one special doctor to whom it was passed was Edward Jenner.

11

AS SOON AS THE DISCUSSION CAME TO AN END, the caretaker and his wife quickly entered the room, walked to a long table and placed on it several trays of food and drink. One tray contained a variety of finger sandwiches made of ham, cheese or cucumber. Another tray bore an assortment of cakes: English pound cake, marble cake, banana cake and walnut cake. In addition, the table also held containers of hot tea and coffee, milk, water and cubes of sugar. At one end of the table, the servants placed small plates, cups and saucers, utensils and cloth napkins. A decanter of Port wine and the appropriate glasses reposed on a separate tray, at the other end. Some of the women would have preferred Sherry wine, but Sherry would have been considered a boorish drink, this late in the evening.

Once the trays were in place and their contents neatly arranged, the caretaker approached Prof and Iris and announced, with great dignity, that the kitchen was closed for the night, and he and his wife would now excuse themselves and retire to their room. He then addressed the professor, even more formally, "Sir, is there anything else that you require this evening?"

"No," the Prof answered hesitantly.

The caretaker then announced, in a loud, clear voice, for all to hear, "Sir, tomorrow morning, breakfast will be served in the breakfast room promptly at eight."

The guests got the message: eight o'clock promptly, or your eggs, toast and coffee will be served cold. Then the caretaker and his wife bid the Prof and Iris, "Good evening" and, deliberately ignoring the guests, marched stiffly out of the room.

Once the caretaker had left, and the Prof was again in charge, he said, "It is time for all of us to take a break and have some refreshments."

The guests sitting on the soft sofas had difficulty getting up, particularly the ladies. The disarming combination of the soft cushions, cold air and lack of activity all contributed to their joints and muscles becoming stiff, and as the guests began to rise, muffled moans and groans were heard. The men were on their feet first, and each of the husbands, in turn, took his wife's hand and assisted her getting up. As each of the wives reached a standing position, she had her own comment, "Oh, it feels so good to move about;" "I'm so stiff my joints creak;" "Dear, I've been sitting much too long. I doubt that I shall be able to walk."

The guests immediately made their way to the great hearth, held their hands to the flames, and rubbed them together vigorously. They then turned their backs toward the fire for just a moment, before heading for the attractively set table that awaited them.

After placing sandwiches and cakes on their plates and filling their cups with hot drinks, they assembled in groups of twos and threes to indulge themselves in idle chatter, as they ate. Eventually, they returned to their original seats, with either a glass of Port wine or a hot drink in their hands.

Prof and Iris assumed their cherished locations close to the fireplace, and the Prof announced, "If you please, ladies and gentlemen," demanding everyone's undivided attention. Then, directly addressing Valerie Jones, Jimmy Jones' wife, he asked her about smallpox in Colonial America, and ended his questioning with, "Of course, by Colonial America, I mean when you were still fortunate enough to belong to the great British Empire. I'm only kidding, Valerie." The comment was made with a wide grin on his face, forehead wrinkled, his eyes partly closed, and the muffled sound of laughter emanating from deep in his throat.

The Prof's jokes were never, ever funny—even though he seemed to think that they were; he did, however, have a quick sense of humor when someone else told a funny story.

Valerie smiled, which exaggerated her lovely facial features and high-lighted her attractive white teeth. Of course, she took no offense to the Prof's attempt at a joke, and she quickly retorted, "I never realized that the American colonies were part of the British Empire. I just assumed that the English troops stationed there were merely tourists, much like the many English people who have taken over Miami Beach these days."

"Very good!" the Prof replied. "Now that that is out of the way, tell us about your Colonial America and smallpox."

"As you know," Valerie began, "smallpox was present in Colonial America almost from the beginning, when the English Puritans founded Plymouth Colony in 1620, and it was that loathsome disease which decimated the Indian tribes of New England, during most of the seventeenth century. The Indians had no immunity, since they never had been exposed to smallpox before, and when they accidentally contracted it from the settlers, the tribes were devastated; in some cases, nearly all who got the disease died. There were, however, other incidents of British troops and the English settlers purposely infecting the Indians with smallpox. Biowarfare, the killing of an enemy by spreading germs, was first used in the American colonies in 1763 by Sir Jeffrey Amherst. He ordered his troops to deliberately spread smallpox among the Indian tribes, by giving them blankets contaminated with pus and scabs, from patients who had succumbed to smallpox. It would seem, however, that the human race hasn't progressed very much, during the past nearly 250 years, except that now we know how to use biowarfare much more efficiently and effectively. I wonder if it is proper to refer to this as progress?"

No one ventured to answer the question, since they assumed that it was merely rhetorical.

Valerie continued, "During the first part of the eighteenth century, Philadelphia and Boston were the foremost colonial cities and names like Benjamin Franklin and the Rev. Cotton Mather were, in their own ways, associated with the disease, smallpox. Franklin's son died of the disease, during the 1753 epidemic. His tombstone and grave can be found, even to this day, within the city limits of Philadelphia.

"Over the years, Boston was beset by recurrent attacks of smallpox, with its most lethal epidemic occurring in 1721. Cotton Mather, a minister, and the first American-born Fellow of the Royal Society, invoked God's help to get the city through the smallpox epidemic, because there was little else that could be done for the sick, save fasting, self-denial, prayer and quarantine. The colonists, without a proper understanding of the disease or how it was spread, knew that isolating a patient with smallpox was one way of preventing its dissemination. However, it was also Cotton Mather who was responsible for introducing smallpox inoculation—or variolation—after learning of its use in England. It was during the 1721 epidemic that Mather had the opportunity to persuade a Dr. Zabdiel Boylston of Boston to perform the first variolations in America, and members of the Mather family were supposedly the first recipients of the procedure in the country.

"Boston was a major port city of nearly 11,000 people, most of whom were young and susceptible to contracting smallpox. Adults, however, tended to be immune to the disease, after having been infected and survived previous epidemics. The 1721 epidemic started when a ship from the Caribbean arrived in the port of Boston with an infected crewman on board. Immediately, the infected seaman was taken into custody and forcibly quarantined in a house close to the docks. In front of the house, a red flag was planted as a warning that within was a person with smallpox. On the flag was printed the following words, 'God have mercy on this house.' But, to no one's surprise, within days, other members of the crew came down with the same disease. Almost without delay, close to a thousand citizens took flight from Boston. Of the nearly six thousand people who were later stricken with the disease, approximately nine hundred, mainly infants and young children, died."

After Valerie finished, the Prof took over, "Having completed his two years with Dr. Hunter, Jenner was anxious to return to Berkeley. Murray, since you spent time in that area of England, perhaps you would like to tell us about Jenner's new life in Berkeley. It certainly must have been quite different from the one he lived in London, with the Hunter family."

While the Prof's remarks to Murray may have sounded like a request, Murray and everyone else knew that the Prof was telling Murray to become active and participate in the discussions.

Murray, in his early fifties, had fine features, wore eyeglasses and had a head of thick, straight brown hair with streaks of gray running through it. Although a South African by birth and a Canadian citizen by necessity—he had to earn a living—Murray was unabashedly a citizen of London by desire. If he had his choice of where to live, he certainly would have selected London, though no one in the group knew why he was such a committed Londoner. Perhaps what he found appealing about London was the ability to exchange ideas freely without fear of retribution.

Murray grew up in South Africa during the apartheid, which he hated, and he had had problems with the government for expressing antiapartheid sentiments, as a young medical student. After being forced out of South Africa by the government, because of his political views against the apartheid, Murray immigrated to England and found work as a medical doctor in London. During the time Murray lived in London, he joined with other South Africans to lecture, and collect money to support the antiapartheid movement back home. Murray frequently spoke emotionally about what he saw as the social and cultural advantages of living in London, advantages that, according to Murray, existed nowhere else in the world.

Murray seemed surprised, when called upon by the Prof to speak. Modest to the extreme, he stammered for a moment, then spoke with a decidedly refined, but high-pitched, Oxford English accent. "Of course, Prof, but before I get on with it, I would like to point out that, at this time in his career, Jenner would have been addressed as Mister and not Doctor, since he had had his early medical training with Mister Ludlow who was a surgeon, and, at that time, Jenner still did not have a university medical degree. So when Jenner returned to Berkeley, he would have been more properly addressed as Mister Jenner, a title used by all surgeons. As a country doctor, Jenner practiced both medicine and surgery, in which case the terms, Mister and Doctor, didn't imply a difference in function. However, ordinarily the term, Doctor, was considered more prestigious. Throughout his career as a physician, Jenner regretted not being able to use the term, Doctor, before his name. Fortunately, because of his acclaimed work with smallpox vaccination, he eventually was awarded an honorary degree of Doctor of Medicine, but this recognition came late in his life."

Murray moved his hands and arms incessantly when lecturing. Possibly, this quirk was caused by the fact that, while he was lecturing, he was unable to smoke. Murray was what you would call a heavy smoker, and the only time he seemed to relax at all was when he had a cigarette in his hand. Prof made no pretense of his dislike of anyone smoking in his house, so it must have taken considerable willpower for Murray to make it through the weekend. He did manage to slip outdoors occasionally, and the rest of the party, all non-smokers, pretended not to notice.

"Thank you, Murray," said Prof, "we all appreciate your reminding us of the difference between the two terms, because it can be confusing at times. Now let's get on with Jenner's return to his home village of Berkeley."

Murray was knowledgeable and could express himself elegantly. However, he always seemed to stutter or stammer, before warming up to his subject. This time was no exception. He took a sip of his wine, shifted in his chair and replied, "Ahhh, fine, Prof. I shall. Back in Berkeley, Jenner was…"

◆ ◆ ◆

Jenner was delighted to be away from London, a city which he vehemently disliked, even though he enjoyed his two years with the Hunters. He was happy to be back in the village of Berkeley, in Gloucestershire, near the Severn River, a country setting that he knew and for which he had deep and tender feelings. Berkeley was not much more than a small collection of humble country dwellings, surrounded by farms and the prodigiously huge Berkeley Castle. It was here that he would be the doctor for all the people, doing work that brought him great pleasure. At heart, Jenner was a homely, unpretentious man, who had no desire to become rich or famous from his work. On the contrary, he felt privileged to be able to conduct himself in the profession of his own choosing. Of course, he needed to earn enough money to one day support a family, but he considered it being unfaithful to his Hippocratic Oath to over-charge a patient. He swore to take care of the sick and look after the poor, and he took that oath seriously.

But there were compensations, other than money, that living in Berkeley provided, and that did not exist in London. In his spare time, he could explore the stretches of lowlands lying between the hills, and walk along the banks of the Severn River, searching for the remains of prehistoric animals that had frequented this rich and beautiful area, millions of years ago. Jenner never lost his inborn tendency to behave in a way characteristic of his nature. As a child, he had explored these same fields studying the natural habitat of the small animals, plants and birds that were so abundant there.

Jenner could not be happier serving the good, solid countryfolk, and away from the desultory and depraved atmosphere that was present in London. Besides, he could no longer abide the pretentious London doctors, whose major goal was to accumulate wealth, and who sold themselves by their patronizing and indulging behavior, rather than their medical or surgical skills. He was determined to bring to the Vale of Berkeley the best of medical care.

It was the spring of 1773, and he had just turned 24 years old, when he arrived in Berkeley. The weather was invigorating, the air smelled sweet and the trees were budding. No longer would he have to be molested by the foul-smelling, contaminated air of London. Immediately, he was popular with the pastoral people for whom he would care. He knew their language, understood their likes and dislikes, and was familiar with their families, farms and farm animals. His popularity stemmed from the warmth of his personality, and his sense of humor, which he shared with them. Their lives were difficult, at times, but they survived the harshness and severity of country living without complaining excessively. Jenner found in them an inner strength, and the practice of looking on the bright side of things, characteristics that were lacking in the poor of London.

Before getting on with serious scientific work, Jenner had first to spend time with his brother, Stephen, whom he hadn't seen in two years. It was Stephen, and of course John Hunter, who had dramatically influenced his life. Oddly enough, these two men had contrasting personalities, still each, in his own way, had a positive influence on Jenner. Stephen by nature was gentle and willing to stay within the bounds of accepted religious teachings; Hunter, on the other hand, acknowledged no restricting limits, based upon medical tradition, and it was this desire for the pursuit of new medical knowledge that Hunter passed on to Jenner. Nevertheless, the principles taught to Edward, as a young boy, by Stephen gave him the tenacity to stand up to and overcome the unpredictable changes and challenges that keep occurring in life. It was Stephen who taught Jenner, above all, to venerate God and to love and respect his family. He explained to him about duty, honor and charity, and what were considered good manners, besides instilling in him an unyielding respect for all women. While Jenner assimilated the distinguishing traits of both Stephen and Hunter, he still maintained his own distinctive personality. He was highly intelligent, quick to learn, determined, sociable and friendly.

But it was as if his reputation as a skilled surgeon preceded him to Berkeley, for within six months after returning home, he had organized a financially successful medical and surgical practice. Jenner's time in London enabled him to become a first-class surgeon, which meant that he operated with speed, dexterity and cleanliness, all the necessary surgical traits that saved patients' lives, at a time when anesthetics and antiseptics were unknown. It would take another century before an acceptable anesthetic was available, and the need for sterile operating conditions was understood.

While he was new to the doctors of Berkeley and the surrounding areas, Jenner was soon accepted by them for his skillful surgery and keen medical judgment. The local surgeons frequently called on him to operate on patients requiring his special surgical skills. Soon his medical and surgical abilities were known and required well beyond the Vale of Berkeley. He was also fortunate because, at one point in his career, his medical and surgical skills were acknowledged by a German University that offered him a degree of Doctor of Physic (Doctor of Medicine). It was an honor that he could ill afford to refuse, but he did so, because his mentor, Dr. Hunter, did not have a comparable academic title.

About this time, Jenner became romantically involved with a young lady who, to his disheartenment, rejected his proposal of marriage. He told all in a letter to Hunter about how his unrequited love left him mournful and melancholy. Hunter, assuming the role of the sympathetic father figure, didn't encourage Jenner's marked disappointment, but took a pragmatic position when he counseled, "I can easily conceive how you must feel, for you have two passions to cope with, namely, being disappointed in love, and being defeated; both will wear out, perhaps the first, the soonest." Hunter, ever the hard-working and persevering scientist, as much as told Jenner, in the last part of his letter, to get over his love affair and to get on with his scientific experiments with the hedgehogs.

Berkeley was best known historically for Berkeley Castle, dating back to the 12th century. One day, in the future, it would become famous as Jenner's birthplace, and the location where he did his scientific studies that led to the use of vaccination as a way of preventing the disease, smallpox. Nevertheless, for Hunter, Berkeley and its surrounding area were merely a geological and biological utopia, and he was constantly entreating Jenner to search out and to send him biological specimens for his collection. Of the many specimens that Jenner would eventually send to him, the one that Hunter cherished was the skeleton of a small whale that had made its way up the Severn River during a high tide. Jenner found the whale, dissected it and sent the skeleton, by coach, to Hunter in London.

Life in Berkeley for Jenner was an equal mixture of the practice of medicine and scientific research. Fortunately, he had an abundance of energy and thus, he was able to do justice to both.

Above all, though, for Jenner, the resolute country doctor, the welfare of his patients was always his primary concern, as was evidenced by a near fatal house-call he was determined to make to a farm one extremely cold, snowy night. The episode is best described by Jenner himself.

"The air felt more intensely cold than I ever remember to have experienced. The ground was deeply covered with snow, and it blew quite a hurricane, accompanied with continual snow. Being well clothed, I did not find the cold made much impression on me till I ascended the hills...There was no possibility of keeping the snow from drifting under my hat, so that half of my face and my neck was, for a long time, wrapt (sic) in ice...I had still two miles to go. As the sense of external cold increased, the heat about the stomach seemed to increase. I had the same sensations as if I had drunk a considerable quantity of wine or brandy; and my spirits rose in proportion to this sensation.

"I felt...like one intoxicated...My hands at last grew extremely painful, and this distressed my spirits in some degree. When I came to the house I was unable to dismount without assistance. I was almost senseless; but I had just recollection and power enough left to prevent the servants from bringing me to a fire...I could bear no greater heat than that of the stable for some time. Rubbing my hands in snow took off the pain quickly. The parts which had been most benumbed, felt for some time as if they had been slightly burnt. My horse lost part of the cuticle and hair at the upper part of the neck, and also from his ears. I had not the least inclination to take wine, or any kind of refreshment."

Jenner was fortunate to have survived this harrowing experience for, on such a night, many a farmer or wayfarer was found frozen to death, huddled in some lonely spot trying to keep warm. His detailed description of hypothermia is one of the earliest on record, and it showed Jenner's astute ability for observing and recording important clinical events, even one that nearly cost his life. During his entire medical career, he continually made original and useful medical observations. His account of hypothermia alerted doctors, for the first time, to the proper treatment for frostbite. He cautioned that the slow warming of a hypothermic individual is imperative, and that too rapid warming of frozen tissues can lead to cell death, blood coagulation and eventually gangrene.

During Jenner's time, there were few medicines of value with which to treat patients. Hunter often lamented that there were only four useful medicines, no matter how many herbs and ointments were displayed in the fancy jars in the apothecary shops. Since medicines of any clinical value were rare, bloodletting, leeching and purging were frequently used to treat diseases. Still, herbal mixtures which were no more than placebos were commonly used. But Jenner possessed, in addition to his surgical skills and good medical judgment, his own, God-given, healing powers which included his self-assured personality and manly appearance.

If a patient lived a great distance away, he was never in a hurry to leave and frequently stayed the night caring for the individual. His company was always welcomed, since he had many stories to tell, and because of his knowledge of the area, he could discuss new methods of farming or gardening. The evenings would conclude with the good doctor reciting one of his poems, for instance *Berkeley Fair:*

> *"The sun drove off the twilight gray,*
> *And promised all a cloudless day;*
> *His yellow beams glanced o'er the dews,*
> *And changed to gems their pearly hues,*
> *The song birds on every spray,* (sic)
> *And sang as if they knew the day;*
> *The blackbird piped his mellow note;*
> *The gold finch strained his downy throat;*
> *The little wren, too, left her nest,*
> *And striving, sang her very best;*
> *The robin wisely kept away,*
> *His song too plaintive for the day*
> *'Twas Berkeley Fair, and nature's smile*
> *Spread joy around for many a mile."*

He was equally enjoyed by the young ladies of the houses where he stayed, since he too was young, agreeable, and reveled in dancing and singing. The evenings were spent with Jenner entertaining the ladies by playing one of his songs on the flute or the violin. Jenner was always the gentleman, and, since he was a bachelor, he was exceptionally discreet and mannerly when in the presence of the young ladies, a trait that remained with him throughout his life.

12

AS THE EVENING PROGRESSED, it began to rain, the temperature fell, and the huge living room was now colder than when the evening began. Even the blazing fire was not enough to compensate for the inclement weather, and Prof knew there was little he could do to make his guests more comfortable. He, therefore, recommended that they put on heavy topcoats or warm sweaters for the remainder of the evening. The ladies acknowledged that they would follow his advice, while each man, in turn, assured Prof that he was adequately dressed. Fortunately, the ladies had made the right decision, because the evening would go on longer than expected. As the discussions proceeded, the room temperature continued to fall, despite the amount of firewood Prof added to the fire, or how vigorously he poked the logs. For the Prof and Iris, things were different; they had been through chilly evenings many times before and they were well prepared. Prof wore a warm vest under his jacket, and Iris had slipped on a thick sweater earlier in the evening, during one of the intervals. Besides, by right of seniority, they had usurped the warmest spots in the room.

Once the ladies returned, blanketed in heavy topcoats, they immediately took their seats and waited for Prof to resume the discussions. Before Prof had a chance to speak, Cedric took over the proceedings. No one was surprised, since Cedric was prone to monopolizing the conversation. Everyone was aware of his aggressive behavior and they were at times resentful, but on this occasion, no one said anything. Cedric began, "Jenner was fortunate to have studied with Hunter for, without his guidance, Jenner, on his own, wouldn't have made any of his remarkable discoveries."

Everyone groaned in unison when they heard such a ridiculous statement. Jimmy was the first to respond. "Cedric, you can't be serious. Hunter may have encouraged Jenner to do research work, in addition to being a country doctor, but that was all. The ideas and hard work were Jenner's."

The Prof, too, was reluctant to let Cedric's remark go unchallenged. "Cedric, the best rebuttal to your observation is that Jenner's greatest discovery, namely cowpox vaccination, was totally his own creation. In fact, on numerous occasions, Jenner told Hunter about dairymaids who had had cowpox and were unable to contract smallpox, and that he wanted to investigate this phenomenon. Hunter discouraged Jenner from following this line of investigation, probably for selfish reasons, considering that for the past several years Jenner had been supplying him with biological samples and animal information, so that he could continue his own research. If Jenner diverted time and energy to the study of smallpox, he would be less attentive to Hunter's needs, or so Hunter thought. Undoubtedly, Hunter wanted Jenner to continue to collect biological samples for the new comparative anatomy museum that he was building.

"No, Cedric, I think that you have it all wrong this time."

Cedric said nothing, even though he felt hurt, but his sour facial expression said it all. He was perturbed and glanced about the room, as if he were searching for support from someone in the group, but it was all in vain.

At this point, the Prof began to detect differences of opinion within the group which could prolong the discussions. An evening that began as a cursory celebration of Jenner's birthday was now turning into a prolonged review of his life.

While the Prof was still thinking about Jenner, Murray commented, "Good old Jenner stirred up lots of controversy in his day, and it would seem this evening is no exception."

Valerie nodded her head in full agreement and added, "Let's examine some of the data before we get caught up in the dilemmas that Jenner had to face in England, during the eighteenth century. Jenner's idea that cowpox vaccination could prevent smallpox was a spanking new concept. There was no basis in medicine for what he wanted to do, namely, take matter from a diseased animal and use it to prevent an entirely different disease in humans. While it doesn't seem outlandish to us, it made no sense to most people, during the eighteenth century. Anytime anyone proposes a new concept in science, and it works, there is bound to be trouble."

The Prof, being somewhat more conservative, added, "That's true, Valerie, but we have to be careful and not too all-inclusive, because there are exceptions to that rule."

"Fine, Prof, I'll accept that," Valerie said.

Sarah picked up on the conversation, "Life for Jenner as a naturalist and a researcher was just beginning. So far, we have learned something about his family and his education, up to the period of his life when he became a doctor. Next, we learned that Hunter turned a simple country doctor into a first-class research scientist. Let's find out what Jenner did with his new training."

"You're right, Sarah." The Prof suggested that she might want to continue along this line of reasoning.

The group unanimously agreed, but with some reluctance on the part of Cedric.

"That's it then," said the Prof. "Why don't you carry on with your comments, Sarah?"

Contrary to her initial reluctance to contribute to the discussions, earlier in the evening, Sarah now was eager to participate.

"At that time…"

◆ ◆ ◆

At that time, major economic and ethical changes were taking place. For example, the seeds of the modern day Industrial Revolution, which had earlier been planted, were just beginning to take root. Water power was driving simple machines and young people were just beginning to leave the farms to find work in the big cities, such as Manchester and London. King George III was on the throne, and the great Prime Minister, William Pitt the younger, who brought about important financial changes in the government, was running the country for the crown. The ethical and moral issues of slavery were being raised and attacked, and soon the religiously inspired politician and antislavery advocate, William Wilberforce, would force it to its natural conclusion. It took time, but Wilberforce and others finally brought the abolition of slavery to the British Empire, in 1833.

Jenner had no difficulty building a successful practice, once he got started; the people of Berkeley had been awaiting his return. They knew him from childhood and respected his family. His father had been their pastor and now his brother, Stephen, was serving their parish. What Jenner quickly learned, when he began practicing medicine in the country, was that there were innumerable diseases that he hadn't encountered during training in London. Fortunately, through his correspondence with Hunter, which was voluminous, he received advice about treating these new diseases. At times, recommendations by Hunter about a patient's diagnosis and treatment were invaluable to Jenner, but this was not always true. For example, Hunter's advice could be soothing without being useful, such as, "Be quiet and think yourself well off that the patient is not dead."

Jenner was popular with the townspeople, since they knew that he genuinely liked and respected everyone. It was not unusual for one or more of his friends, who enjoyed his conversations, to ride with him during his visits to patients in the surrounding villages and towns.

Jenner became a familiar figure, as he rode on his rounds. He was judged to be a meticulous dresser and usually made house-calls wearing a blue coat with yellow buttons, tan buckskins, highly polished jockey boots with silver spurs attached at the heels, a broad-brimmed hat, and he carried a silver-handled whip.

To add to the intellectual environment of the community, Jenner became a founding member of two important scientific clubs, whose members held their meetings at local taverns or inns. It was at these meetings that pertinent medical topics were discussed.

While the early part of the evenings was used for the exchange of intellectual information, as the evenings wore on, there was music, as well as songs and the recitation of poems. During these sessions, Jenner was usually the most active participant. He recited his own poetry and sang songs he had composed. In addition, he contributed to the merriment by playing the flute or the violin. Frequently the evenings ended with everyone in a frolicsome mood, brought on by the excessive use of alcohol, mainly ale or gin.

About this time, an interesting incident took place which revealed something of Jenner's personality and intellectual abilities. While dining with a large party, the question arose whether the temperature was highest in the center of the flame of a candle, or at some small distance above the top of the flame. Among the various guests, opinions differed, but Jenner, with his usual ingenuity and inventiveness, quickly settled the dispute. Placing the candle before him, he inserted a finger into the center of the flame and was able to leave it there for several seconds. Next, he put his finger a little above the tip of the flame and was immediately forced to remove the finger. "There, gentlemen," he observed, "the question is settled."

Attending the party was a gentleman who had a sizable measure of political influence, and who marveled at Jenner's talent and good sense. The following day, he sought out Jenner and offered him an appointment in the East Indies at a substantial compensation. Of course, Jenner refused, but thanked him for his offer of such a generous emolument to work at the highly reputable post.

It was not long after Jenner left London that he received a letter from Hunter offering him the opportunity to become a partner at his school and participate with him is his research. The school that Hunter had started quickly became successful, and along with his surgical duties at the hospital and his commitment to establishing a comparative anatomy museum, he needed help. Hunter had respect for Jenner as a physician, naturalist and research scientist and he, therefore, offered him a partnership. As part of the partnership agreement, Hunter wanted Jenner to pay a thousand pounds, which was reasonable for such a prestigious position. Without delay, Jenner wrote back to Hunter thanking him for the offer, and explained to him that he had no intention of leaving Berkeley. Jenner could easily have raised the thousand pounds; however, he enjoyed his life in Berkeley, and he knew that he would never be happy living in London.

Once Hunter accepted the fact that Jenner would not be joining him, he returned to his old ways of urgently requesting biological specimens from Jenner. They were both interested in studying the cuckoo bird, and Hunter wanted Jenner to supply him with a cuckoo nest with an egg in it. Since it was winter, Jenner could not satisfy his request.

Animal hibernation, the act of an animal sleeping through the winter, was another one of Hunter's concerns, and he wished to use the hedgehog as his experimental animal. Hedgehogs were plentiful in Berkeley, and Jenner was able to supply Hunter with these animals. The hedgehogs were put into Hunter's garden where they could be studied during hibernation. Unfortunately, all the animals either died or were eaten by scavengers.

At this juncture, Hunter had to rely on Jenner to perform the necessary experiments in Berkeley. He wrote to Jenner specifying what tests he wanted done. The thermometer had recently been introduced into scientific research work, and Hunter, luckily, was able to furnish Jenner with one of these new instruments for the hibernation studies.

Jenner was instructed to locate a hibernating hedgehog, on a cold day, and pass the thermometer into the anus of the animal and record the temperature. Following this, he was to cut a small hole in its belly and pass the thermometer up by the liver and again record its temperature. Jenner made a series of these readings over the winter on numerous hedgehogs. Finally, Jenner was to examine hedgehog nests, to determine how well they were protected from the cold, and ascertain if the animals stored food in the nests for the winter. Jenner, likewise, had to record the weights of the hedgehogs, before and after hibernation.

Later on, Hunter who was a member of the Royal Society, presented his hibernation studies at one of their meetings, and he was richly acclaimed for this work. Jenner also wrote a paper on hedgehogs which, for whatever reason, he never published. The report was found with his papers after he died.

Because its reproduction cycle was an enigma, the cuckoo bird was a legitimate subject for study. Both Hunter and Jenner were interested in cuckoo birds. Since cuckoos were plentiful in the Vale of Berkeley, during the mating season, Hunter encouraged Jenner to study the reproductive cycle of these birds.

Cuckoos start arriving in Berkeley about the middle of April, to reproduce. The birds do not pair, since the female is promiscuous and will mate with many different males. After mating, the female deposits her eggs in the nests of other birds and leaves the area. Theoretically such a reproductive cycle, where both the eggs and the chicks go unattended, should lead to the extinction of the cuckoo bird. But that never happened.

Within the hedgerows of Berkeley, many different species of small birds built their nests and laid their eggs. Jenner was able to place a hedge sparrow's nest near the edge of a hedgerow, where he could see clearly what was happening. Jenner observed numerous female cuckoos laying their eggs in the nests of hedge sparrows, alongside the hedge sparrow eggs. What happened next, as he observed the nests, was totally unexpected. First, the hedge sparrow female accepted the cuckoo's eggs, along with her own clutch of eggs, to be incubated. The cuckoo eggs and the hedge sparrow eggs were about the same size, even though the cuckoo grows to be a much larger bird than the hedge sparrow.

The hedge sparrow mother incubated the cuckoo eggs, which usually hatched earlier than her own eggs. Shortly after hatching, the cuckoo chick sought out a hedge sparrow's egg or chick and ejected it from the nest. And the method of ejection was quite amazing, too. The cuckoo chick maneuvered the hedge sparrow egg or chick onto its back, using its rump and wings to secure it there. With the egg or chick seated in an indentation on the back of the cuckoo chick, near its tail, the cuckoo chick then moved backwards up the side of the nest, until it reached the top, where, with one quick jerk, it ejected its burden from the nest. Afterwards, the cuckoo chick rested and examined its rump with the tip of its wings, to be certain that it had got rid of its victim. After the cuckoo chick was convinced that the hedge sparrow egg or chick was gone, it fell back into the nest.

The hedge sparrow mother accepted the cuckoo chick as her own, feeding it and tending to it needs. Jenner verified his observations by drawing a picture of a female hedge sparrow, in her nest, feeding a cuckoo chick that was almost twice her size.

Hunter presented Jenner's findings at a meeting of the Royal Society. Many members received Jenner's story about the habits of young cuckoo chicks with disbelief and contempt. In spite of this, Jenner was honored for this work by being elected a fellow of the Royal Society.

Later, antivaccinationists used his conclusions about the cuckoo bird, as a means of refuting his conclusions about vaccination preventing smallpox. They claimed that if he was mistaken about the breeding habits of the cuckoo bird, he must also be mistaken about his claims for vaccination.

For years, some naturalists rejected Jenner's conclusions about the cuckoo chick's ability to eject eggs and chicks from a nest. But gradually Jenner's work was corroborated. Oddly enough, it took 140 years before the ejection process was photographed, verifying Jenner's initial observations.

Jenner's cuckoo bird studies continued, and, over the years, developed into a much larger study of the migratory habits of many different species of birds. This work was continued for the rest of his life, and was interrupted only during his intensive investigations leading to the discovery that vaccination prevented smallpox.

Jenner's large body of work as a naturalist is overshadowed by the overwhelming success of his discovery of vaccination as a method of preventing smallpox. When Jenner did his experiments with the cuckoo bird, he was merely following the edict that he so often heard from Hunter: "But why think about it? Why not try the experiment?" As a young boy, Jenner began his life's work as a naturalist collecting the nests of dormice, and finished his life as a naturalist characterizing the migratory habits of birds.

13

"LIFE IN THE EIGHTEENTH CENTURY was decidedly different from what it is today," said Valerie.

The Prof was quick to respond, since he realized that to properly understand Jenner, it was important to place him in his own century. "Yes, you're right Valerie. If we were somehow able to physically revert to the eighteenth century, it would be like visiting another country, for the speech would be different, as would the customs and mores. Perhaps, it would be helpful for us to stop and consider what was happening during the eighteenth century."

Cedric, always ready to be negative, interrupted. "You can't. It's impossible. Why even try?"

Prof liked to describe Cedric's negativity as coming from a person who, "thinks nothing is ever good, only sometimes it is worse." So he gave him a sideways glance of disapproval and ignored his remark.

Jimmy, on the other hand, was inclined to hope for the best. "Let's do it, so long as we don't get bogged down in all the nuances of that century. It is difficult enough to make sense of all the events of our own century."

"Good for you Jimmy," commented Sarah. "I think that somewhat more knowledge about the workings of the eighteenth century will give us additional insight into what it was like for Jenner, both as a doctor and a research scientist." Sarah's remark contradicted her husband, Cedric's, earlier statement, to some extent, so she hesitated to look towards him for approval.

"Fine Sarah, suppose you get us started," the Prof immediately suggested.

Sarah accepted the challenge, even though it would further antagonize Cedric. "Let's see, now. During the latter part of the eighteenth century, King George III, the mad king, was on the throne. His wildly excited and disorderly behavior was documented in a movie entitled, "The Madness of King George." During his reign, some thought that the King was just plain crazy, while others, in deference to his being the King, were more inclined to explain away his bizarre behavior as being odd, unconventional or just out of the ordinary. Only years later, in the twentieth century, when our biochemical and genetic knowledge made major advances, was it possible to correctly diagnose the true cause of the poor King's mental illness. The unfortunate and much maligned King had a rare genetic disease called porphyria, as the underlying cause of his intermittent episodes of odd and unconventional behavior. Porphyrins are purple-red pigments found in every cell in the body, and their presence in the hemoglobin of red blood cells gives them their red coloring.

"Porphyria is caused by a chemical disturbance in the utilization of the body's porphyrins. The King was suffering from intermittent porphyria, and during an attack, he showed evidence of disturbed behavior and was wrongly diagnosed as being mad or insane. Porphyria has an autosomal dominant mode of transmission, so that one abnormal gene was enough to cause the King's abnormal physical and mental problems.

King George III was America's last king, and his life-span closely coexisted with that of Jenner's. The King was born in June of 1738 and he died in January of 1820. The poor chap had five separate lingering episodes of madness; at times, the attacks were so bad that he had to be put in a strait-jacket. His first attack occurred when he was 27 years old, and he died during his fifth attack, when he was age 82.

The renowned American jurist, Oliver Wendell Homes, wrote a little ditty about odd ancestors that seems to fit here. It goes:

> "We are all omnibuses in which our ancestors
> ride, and every now and then one of them sticks
> his head out and embarrasses us."

Perhaps, like a lot of other families, King George had many odd and disturbed ancestors; they, most likely, didn't have porphyria though. Dr. Jenner certainly knew the King, had audiences with him and was admired by both the King and the Queen. Near the end of his life, Jenner was appointed Physician Extraordinary to King George IV. Jenner was very old by then and not well, so it was an honorary appointment, without any real responsibilities.

"Early in the century, the prime minister was William Pitt the Elder. It was he who united the English and the Scots, forming what we call today the British Empire. Later, William Pitt the Younger became prime minister at the tender age of 24, and imposed fiscal discipline and sensible accounting practices on the Empire. At the same time, the America colonies were having their own problems with England—but let's not rehash the Revolutionary War. The Industrial Revolution was just beginning and the mechanization of spinning cotton and wool was a big part of the early movement. Watt invented the steam engine; Cavendish discovered hydrogen; and Priestley discovered oxygen. These were all important discoveries in science."

"You are right, but don't forget Davy discovered nitrous oxide or, as it is known today, laughing gas," Murray commented.

Sarah continued, "The eighteenth century culture embraced new scientific discoveries, and interest in science filtered down from the King through all levels of society. Science lectures and demonstrations were frequent and were well attended by the general public.

"It was fashionable for wealthy gentlemen to do their own experiments, and collect biological specimens. They also used rain gauges and made meteorological measurements to keep track of the weather. These enlightened men used their own money, time and energy to scientifically describe or appraise natural events, circumstances or experiences that were apparent to their senses. Some of their efforts to establish scientific principles or truths were esoteric science and had no immediate practical value; still, there were those whose research had immediate and useful applications. One of those outstanding eighteenth century scientists, whose research had immediate and beneficial application, was Dr. Jenner."

Not to be left out of the discussion, Ruth quickly remarked, "We should mention some important writers who were contemporaries of Jenner, such as, Boswell, Burns, Byron and Goethe; and let's not forget the irritable and irascible Englishman, Samuel Johnson. There are so many good stories circulating about him, even to this day. The one that I like best happened shortly after he finished writing his pivotal English language dictionary. Of course, he was quite a celebrity after that, and on this occasion, he was invited to a dinner party at the home of a rich matron, to commemorate his newly acknowledged triumph. As Johnson entered the house, he was effusively greeted by the matron who made glowing remarks about his new dictionary. After she was finished glorifying Johnson, and acting as if he were some sort of god, she sadly commented, "I found an error in the definition of one of the words in your dictionary! I couldn't believe that such a highly intelligent man as you could make such a simple mistake. How could that happen?" Johnson stared directly at her and sarcastically replied, "Stupidity madam, pure stupidity!"

"To prevent us from getting bogged down in so many different social and cultural things that occurred during the eighteenth century, let's limit ourselves. Any suggestions?" queried the Prof.

"Why not limit ourselves to the customs of marriage during Jenner's time?" Valerie replied.

To push the discussion along, the Prof responded, "Excellent, Valerie. Since it was your idea, suppose you get the subject started.

"Fine," Valerie said. "During the eighteenth century, for both royalty and the very wealthy, marriage was an expensive undertaking. A man's wealth determined when it was possible for him to take a bride. English custom dictated that the oldest son in the family inherited everything, upon the death of the senior progenitor. The younger son was left nothing and lived by the generosity of his older sibling. This income then determined at what age he could afford to take a wife.

The youngest son, with no fortune of his own, usually married at about the age of thirty, and his wife would be about ten years younger. For practical purposes, though, they would be of equal social status. A man of wealth or high position, on the other hand, was able to select a wife much younger than he. The richer and more socially prominent the husband, usually the younger was his wife.

"Those at the bottom of the economic scale, wishing to marry, were not restricted by such rigid rules, and in many cases, common and church laws were flouted because of the inability of the man to pay for a marriage license. Thus, clandestine marriages were improvised for the convenience of the marrying couple.

"The Church of England laid down the rules of marriage around 1604. Marriage ceremonies were supposed to be performed publicly, in the parish church of one of the parties, after the banns had been read on three consecutive Sundays. As a way of getting around church law, a man could obtain a marriage license bearing an approved government stamp, from an ecclesiastical administrator to whom he paid a fee. In a third of all marriages, because of the expenses, the couples ignored the law and improvised their own marriage ceremonies. Of course, Jenner's marriage to Catharine Kingscote would have adhered to the canon laws of the Church of England."

"Prof, a remarkable event took place during the century which indirectly involved Jenner getting married," Murray commented.

"Fine, Murray. If it is important you must tell us," the Prof replied.

Murray nodded and began.

"The Montgolfier brothers were..."

◆   ◆   ◆

The Montgolfier brothers were the first to invent and eventually demonstrate the fire balloon in France, in November of 1782. The balloon was three feet in diameter, held 35 cubic feet of heated air, and was made of silk. Unfortunately, after it was launched, there was no way of keeping the air inside the balloon heated, so the flight was limited. But it flew, however, and was a tremendous success. The brothers received enthusiastic approval from all over Europe, but especially in England, where the event was recognized as a major scientific breakthrough.

The brothers solved the problem of sustained flight, by adding a frame to the bottom of the balloon which held a fire that heated the air inside of the balloon, making the balloon a much more effective flying machine. This second balloon was known as a "fire balloon," and variations of it became very popular with the public everywhere. The final culmination of the brother's success came, a year later, when the first manned balloon flight took place over Paris, where an enthusiastic crowd of half a million people were on hand to watch. Present also were the King, Marie Antoinette, and most of the aristocracy of France.

Shortly after the Montgolfier brothers' successful launching of the manned balloon using heated air, Jacques Charles launched a manned balloon using hydrogen. The news of these manned balloon flights quickly spread to other countries, where they were greeted with overwhelming amazement.

The Montgolfier brothers' experiments in balloon flights attracted the attention of scientific men everywhere, including Jenner. He was immediately enthralled by the new invention, and resolved to demonstrate this new form of "aerial navigation," as it was called, to his neighbors in Berkeley. He questioned whether the lifting power of the Montgolfier fire balloon was due to the hot air or the smoke. This was a reasonable scientific question to ask, based upon the lack of knowledge that existed at that time. Regardless of this, however, Jenner elected to launch a balloon using hydrogen gas.

Anxious to repeat the initial, unmanned, scientific achievement of the Frenchmen, Jenner enlisted the help of the Earl of Berkeley and a friend, Edward Gardner, a literary man and a famous poet, to build a balloon. The balloon was constructed in the great hall at Berkeley Castle and was filled with hydrogen gas. It is not known how they produced the hydrogen gas that filled the balloon; however, hydrogen gas was readily available to them, since it previously had been discovered by the English chemist, Cavendish.

The balloon was taken out into the Castle meadow where it gently sailed over the hilly barrier surrounding the vale, making Jenner one of the early balloonists in England. A mild westerly wind carried the balloon for an amazing ten miles, where it landed, without damage, in a meadow a short distance away from Kingscote Park, the home of Jenner's future wife, Catharine Kingscote. Jenner and his friend, Edward Gardner, rode their horses ten miles to retrieve their balloon. When Jenner arrived, he was persuaded by the Kingscote family to have the second launching of the balloon from Kingscote Park. It was on that occasion that he met Catharine Kingscote, and it wasn't long thereafter that he asked her to marry him. Catharine accepted his proposal; however, the marriage didn't take place for several years.

No mention of the size of the balloon is found in any of the records of the flight, but it was thought to be a very small balloon. The second launching of the balloon from Kingscote Park, was also a great success, both as a source of scientific achievement and entertainment as well. The launching of the balloon was attended by the Kingscote family, and just about all the local gentry. Stylish young men and women came charging over the meadow just to touch the balloon, as well as to ask all sorts of silly questions. From miles around, everyone, from the wealthy gentry to the humblest farmer and his family, attended the second launching of Jenner's hydrogen gas balloon. Just before the balloon finally lifted off on its second voyage, Mr. Gardner attached to the balloon, a poem that he had written for the occasion. The poem was quite long and, for whatever reason, contained many romantic stanzas.

The possibility of floating heavy bodies in the atmosphere had been anticipated by scientists for some time, but it took the Montgolfier brothers to invent a method for doing it.

As Jenner was nearing his fortieth birthday, he was now ready to forgo his bachelor days and settle down to married life. Only Jenner knows the reasons that he elected to marry Catharine Kingscote, from a village some ten miles away from Berkeley. But one thing is certain; the marriage was a happy and successful one.

Catharine's facial features were plain but nicely shaped; her skin was like alabaster, especially smooth and white. Her hair was fair in color and complemented her deep blue eyes. She was neither thin nor plump but well formed. She exuded joy and inner stability that made up for what she may have lacked in physical winsomeness. She was one of those fortunate people who possessed qualities that attracted and delighted others. It was as if any action or gesture on her part assumed some magical power, and Jenner was fortunate to have found, so late in life, a wife with so many wonderful qualities and who proved to be a compatible partner. They were married on March 6, 1788.

But there was more to Catharine than just her inner charm. Above all, she could point with pride to being a descendant of a niece of William the Conqueror, and she also had familial connections to the Earl of Berkeley and his family. Moreover, Catharine was favored with a fine dowry which was beneficial to Jenner but certainly not an essential ingredient for his marrying Catharine.

Before Jenner married Catharine, Jenner's religious values were being separated into parts by those people for whom he had the highest respect. In the beginning, Stephen, his brother, who was also a minister, taught him right from wrong, based upon the principles of the Anglican Church. These were religious principles and practical values that enabled him to get through the early years of his life without difficulty.

Back in London, as he entered manhood, he was introduced to religious ideas, by Hunter and his liberal-minded friends, that were, at times, at odds with what he learned as a young boy in Berkeley. Hunter, himself, was not a profoundly pious man; however, he still possessed all the ethical and moral ideals to be classified a righteous individual. He also had his weaknesses: he was short tempered and was loathed to suffer fools. Jenner, too, was changing, for he had difficulty accepting all the religious concepts that he learned from his brother, Stephen. For example, he began to question things that he learned in the Bible's Chapter One of Genesis, which seemed particularly unreasonable to him.

During his London years, he learned about the licentious behavior and questionable moral standards of eighteenth century English royalty which, nevertheless, were not very different from the moral standards of the French and other European royalty. On his return to Berkeley, he had firsthand knowledge of what previously had been only rumors of royal libertine behavior: the Earl of Berkeley had his mistress living at Berkeley Castle.

Fortunately for Jenner, Catharine ruled the family and set the religious concepts to be followed. For Catharine, there were no shades of gray, only right and wrong. The rearing of the children was left in her capable hands. In spite of her moral rigidity, she was known to be both tender and considerate, characteristics indispensable to a happy home and loving marriage. But when it came to the immoral behavior of the Earl, Catharine wasn't so forgiving.

If Catharine had a liability, it was her health. She had been an invalid for some time before their marriage, and except for a brief period during their marriage, she was never known to be robust. In the beginning, her health never seemed to be an impediment, since what she lacked in energy she made up for with her resourcefulness. The first Sunday school in Berkeley was organized and run by her. She bore her first child, a son, without difficulty, within ten months of their marriage. Later, she would give birth, without difficulty, to two more healthy children, another son and a daughter. But it wasn't too long before poor health markedly restricted her social activities.

After their marriage, Jenner bought a home in Berkeley, called Chantry House, that he would refer to in jest as "the cottage." It was, however, much more than a cottage because, in reality, it was a two-storied brick house with some fifteen rooms. It was ideally located close to the village church and Berkeley Castle. From the large front widows, the church and its steeple could be seen as rising out of the church's graveyard and extending above a cluster of lovely trees. At the rear of the house were offices, and a stable where Catharine had a pair of excellent horses and a fine coach, cared for by a groom and a coachman. Servants, in adequate numbers, staffed the house. The garden had a sheltered path where Catharine could walk and still be within sight of Jenner as he looked out his study window. The path led to a grouping of shrubs and trees designed by Jenner to evoke a feeling of seclusion and mystery. In this cloistered area, a neighbor built a small cottage for Jenner, with the intention of giving the garden a rural appearance. Jenner described the cottage as a "retreat for a 'faun,' a satyr, or a deity having the body of a man but with horns, pointed ears, a tail and the hind legs of a goat, or a 'dryad,' a wood nymph." It was all very romantic and mysterious. In later years, the rustic one-room cottage served a less mysterious purpose, when it was used as the place where Jenner attended the hundreds of patients who came to him to be vaccinated.

The rooms in the main house were tastefully decorated in a fashion worthy of a wife who could claim a relationship to the year 1066 and William the Conqueror. The kitchen was plain and unpretentious, and Jenner's wine closet contained five or six different brands which were said to be of rare vintage and excellent flavor.

It was January of 1789 when the happily married couple had their first born son, Edward, named after his father. Jenner was so pleased with the infant that he posted a short note to a friend, Reverend John Clinch, a medical missionary living in Newfoundland, and whose son was also named Edward: "As it is uppermost in my thoughts I must in the first place tell you that I have a son. My dear Catharine has lain in about a fortnight. The child, though small, appears to be remarkably healthy, and I ardently hope that there may as much affection subsist between the young Edwards as between their fathers. There will be no room for more."

Besides his rural practice, Jenner was responsible for the health and well being of the Earl and his family at Berkeley Castle. Catharine had, on occasion, been a guest at the Castle, before her marriage. It was shortly after Edward and Catharine moved into their new home, that the Earl took a mistress and moved her into the Castle. Catharine was unable to reconcile the Earl's behavior with her own strict religious principles, and she openly disapproved of what the Earl had done. In addition, she vehemently refused to visit the castle. It was an honorable gesture, but one that strained the friendly relationship between Jenner and the Earl.

Catharine's health continued to be a problem, and Jenner would pass it off by saying, "She was a woman of the hills and was not vigorous when away from them." But there was more to Catharine's poor health than mere location. Actually, Berkeley, surrounded by low-lying fields and close to the Severn Estuary, was not a good environment for a person with tubercular tendencies, which better explains Catharine's chronic, life-long disability.

Unfortunately, Jenner's oldest son, Edward, was always sickly, and he died of tuberculosis in 1810, at the early age of twenty-one. Robert, the second son, was robust like his father. He attended Exeter College at Oxford, after which he entered the army and attained the rank of colonel. Jenner's daughter, Catharine, named after her mother, took care of her father, after her mother died in 1815. Before he died, in 1823, she married a solicitor and moved to another part of England.

While Jenner enjoyed working and living in Berkeley, his financial requirements forced him to expand his medical practice elsewhere. Jenner received a letter that his nephew, a doctor who recently finished studying with Hunter, was planning on joining him in his medical practice in Berkeley. Jenner realized that the Berkeley medical practice could not support two families, so he elected to set up a second practice for himself in the town of Cheltenham.

Cheltenham was known as a health resort, because of its mineral springs. The practice of bathing in and drinking the mineral waters was reputed to have healing powers. A visit to the spa by King George III for the treatment of his "attacks of madness" stimulated a growing interest in the spa by members of the court and wealthy individuals. Jenner knew that the presence of his Majesty and the royal household at the spa would increase the size of the population of Cheltenham, and there would be a need for additional medical services.

Jenner was a Fellow of the Royal Society and qualified to use the initials FRS after his name, but if he were to be successful in Cheltenham, he needed to have a Doctor of Medicine degree, which would entitle him to be addressed as Doctor Jenner, instead of Mister Jenner. As fortune would have it, two of Jenner's medical colleagues recommended him as a recipient for the degree of Doctor of Medicine from the University of St. Andrew in Scotland, and the degree was awarded him. The awarding of an advanced degree to a qualified individual was a common practice at some universities during the eighteenth century.

14

AS THE EVENING PROGRESSED, THE DAMPNESS of the room penetrated the heavy topcoats of the three women who had been sitting so long on the couch. The logs in the fireplace, by now, were nothing but glowing, hot ashes; but even when the logs were blazing, they did little more than heat the sitting area in the immediate vicinity of the fireplace hearth. Still the smoldering embers did project a visual image of heat. Of course, sitting so long, without moving, undoubtedly contributed more to the ladies' stiffness than did the lack of warmth.

The Prof suggested that everyone get up for a few minutes and move around. With that, the guests were out of their seats, on their feet, and in short order, they formed a semicircle in front of the fireplace, watching as the Prof placed three big logs on top of the glowing cinders. The guests were fascinated watching the Prof, as he poked and pushed the smoldering remains of the fire, teasing and coaxing it to start blazing anew.

Once the group was confident that the Prof had the fire under his control, they began looking for food. Unfortunately, there was little left on the trays, except for cold, stale coffee and tea, leftover wine, and bits and pieces of dried-out sandwiches and end-pieces of cakes. Food, any food, at this hour, was treasured and not to be wasted. After the last morsel was eaten, Valerie remembered that she had a large box of chocolates in her room, which she had intended to give to the Prof and Iris, as a present. Valerie charged out of the room and returned with the box of chocolates, which she handed to Iris, who immediately shared it with everyone.

As usual, the Prof was gracious and suggested, "We are all beholden to Valerie, and we owe her a debt of gratitude, for without her generous present, I doubt that we could have continued."

The standard "Hear, hear!" was the response from the group.

From his self-assigned post at the fireplace, the Prof directed the conversation back to Jenner. "Let's see, we know that Hunter developed a serious illness that eventually led to his death. Murray, since this is going to be a medical discussion, perhaps you would be good enough to enlighten us."

As usual, Prof's request amounted to an order, so Murray was quick to reply. "Right, Prof." Murray took a few seconds to get his thoughts in order.

"Jenner received a letter from Hunter saying that he saw Jenner's brother, Stephen, and that, 'Not two hours after I saw your brother, I was taken ill.' In his letter to Jenner, Hunter never gave any indication of the nature of his illness, but he did say that it was ten days before he could lift his head from the pillow.

"Jenner knew that Hunter would not stay in bed for ten days, unless he was extremely ill. His symptoms and the extended time in bed did not bode well for Hunter. He wrote Jenner that he was going to the city of Bath to rest, and asked Jenner to visit him there. It was not surprising that Hunter elected to go to Bath; after all, it was the most celebrated spa in England. Undoubtedly, Hunter didn't go to Bath in search of a medical remedy for his illness; he was too clever a physician to believe that drinking mineral water would produce a miraculous cure for a serious illness. However, the surroundings were peaceful and relaxing, and besides it was a convenient place to meet his many important friends. Hunter, himself, was by this time one of the most distinguished physicians in England.

"Bath is a wonderful old city dating back to the Roman conquest of England."

Always willing to be helpful, even when not required to do so, Cedric was quick to point out, "Yes, and the Romans remained here for four hundred years. Don't you think that we are spending too much time on Jenner, perhaps, giving him more attention than he deserves?"

"Thank you Cedric." Murray was always forgiving, even of the most boorish remarks, and continued with his story, not anxious to start an unnecessary debate with Cedric. Murray was cognizant of Cedric's frequent surly remarks, which were usually in response to someone else's success.

Murray continued, "The Romans were obsessed with cleanliness and their bath houses were ubiquitous; they went to great extremes to move fresh water into their town, but they never were able to duplicate the monumental aqueducts of Latin Europe. Their sewage systems were the finest for their time, and they were not really duplicated in England, until as late as the nineteenth century.

"Bath, in Roman times was a tiny town called Aquae Sulis. The heart of it was a sacred spring pumping a quarter of a million gallons of mineral water a day, registering at a temperature of 120 degrees F, or 49 degrees C. The Romans used the water to develop thermal baths surrounded by Roman temples.

"Aquae Sulis was lost to antiquity, once the Romans left England, but fortunately the baths were reestablished in 1702 and Bath became the most celebrated spa in England. By the time Hunter went there to rest, the spa was catering to English Royalty and others among the rich and the famous.

"Jenner rode to Bath to see his old friend. It was their first meeting in nearly five years; however, during those years they carried on a two-way correspondence that was both plentiful and productive.

"The reunion for Jenner was not a happy one...."

◆   ◆   ◆

The reunion for Jenner was not a happy one, which it should have been for two old friends. Hunter contended that he was entirely well.

However, to Jenner's experienced eye, it was only too obvious that Hunter was seriously ill and the waters of Bath were of no value to him. Jenner remained silent about Hunter's illness, and only spoke about the pleasant experiments that they jointly worked on, during the past five years.

They talked of many things, but Hunter was interested in hearing about the Freemartin cows which Jenner had previously described to him in a letter. For Hunter, a Freemartin cow was something new, whereas Jenner had occasionally experienced this biological aberration and had actually dissected a number of these animals. A Freemartin is an imperfectly developed female calf, usually sterile, born as the twin of a male. The female calf is masculinized in utero. Jenner went on to describe the unusual changes in the external and internal genital organs of these animals. He finished his little lecture by commenting, "These animals tend to be gentle and do not disturb the other animals in the herd." Hunter acknowledged that it was the first time that he had known of such an animal. In spite of that, at a later date, he lectured before the Royal Society describing these masculinized female cows, based on what he had learned from Jenner.

Jenner then told Hunter about his publication of a new method for preparing Emetic Tartar, a medication of uncertain value for producing vomiting, in an age when overeating and excessive use of alcohol were common practices. As frequently happened during his life, Jenner was ahead of the curve in his scientific thinking. He realized there was a need for the purification and standardization of many of the medicines then being used. As an example, tartaric acid, in its impure form, was being used as Emetic Tartar to induce vomiting in patients; nevertheless, when the medicine was used for this purpose, it was totally unreliable. It was, therefore, impossible to know if too much or too little of the medicine was being used in any given patient. Considering that Emetic Tartar was an insoluble substance containing many impurities, it was no wonder then that a standardized dose could not be determined. Jenner discovered that Emetic Tartar could be purified by recrystallization, enabling him to determine what dosage was required to produce vomiting in a particular patient, and this made the substance safer for the patient to use. His recrystallization method was published as a small pamphlet, at his expense, and was given freely to any doctor requesting it.

Perhaps by coincidence, a hundred years later, the great French scientist, Louis Pasteur, who so much admired and respected Jenner, began his early scientific career doing experiments with tartaric acid crystals. Pasteur discovered that tartaric acid was a mixture of two kinds of crystals which he separated out as mirror images of each other.

It should be noted that Jenner's discovery of vaccination, as a means for preventing smallpox, was essential to Pasteur's own thinking that led to the development of his immunization against rabies.

So many new discoveries were made in chemistry, during the eighteenth century, that it was a turning point in the history of science, and Jenner made his own contribution with his purification of Emetic Tartar.

As much as he tried to pass off his malady as being due to the physical changes associated with aging, Hunter was a chronically ill man, and Jenner knew it. Following careful questioning and examination, Jenner diagnosed his good friend as having angina pectoris, with underlying coronary artery disease. It was a condition which, Jenner realized, eventually would be fatal. Failing to see what purpose it would serve, Jenner elected to remain silent about his diagnosis, in the hope that Hunter would not worry and would be able to continue with his research. It was an unhappy experience for a doctor, any doctor, to know that his best friend was suffering from an incurable disease.

Jenner was pleased to see Hunter again, and to spend time with him, but he left Bath knowing that his mentor, Hunter, was suffering from angina pectoris, a serious disease of the coronary vessels of the heart that, one day, would suddenly kill him.

Angina pectoris is a heart condition that Jenner understood well, since he was the first doctor to demonstrate that the chest pain, called angina pectoris, was associated with a thickening of the walls of the coronary arteries, obstructing the flow of blood. It was a disease that had grave consequences that would eventually lead to death.

Jenner knew that he had made an important clinical discovery, but he restrained any impulse to publish his observations, for fear that Hunter would find out and would despair for his future. But, after Hunter died, a medical colleague of Jenner published a note of Jenner's discovery, along with his own observations on angina pectoris and coronary artery disease.

It was while working with Hunter in London that Jenner saw his first dissection of a patient who had died of angina pectoris. A Dr. Heberden had asked Hunter to do a dissection on such a patient. It was of interest that Dr. Heberden was the first to coin the name, angina pectoris, for severe chest pain in such patients. The dissection was completed without the coronary arteries having been examined by Hunter for, at the time, there was no known association between angina pectoris and coronary artery disease.

Later, while in Berkeley, Jenner came across a patient who had died during an attack of angina pectoris. The patient's doctor asked Jenner to do a dissection, in search of the cause of death. Having found nothing to explain the patient's sudden demise, Jenner decided to make a transverse cut across the base of the heart, and as Jenner explained it, "…when my knife struck against something so hard and gritty as to notch it. I well remember looking up to the ceiling, which was old and crumbling, conceiving that some plaster had fallen down. But, on a further scrutiny, the real cause appeared: the coronaries (arteries) were become bony canals…" It was then that he began to realize that the cause of the angina pectoris and the sudden death were due to a blockage of the blood in the coronary arteries of the heart.

Sometime later, a similar case came to his attention. Once more, another doctor had a patient who died of angina pectoris, and Jenner was asked to do the dissection. As Jenner tells it: "Previous to our examination (dissection) of the body, I offered him (the patient's doctor) a wager that we should find the coronary arteries ossified (bony). This, however proved not to be exactly true; but the coats of the arteries were hard, and a sort of cartilaginous (gristly) canal was formed within the cavity of each artery and there attached, so however, as to be separable as easily as the finger from a tight glove." It was at that time that Jenner was convinced that the obstruction of the coronary arteries was the cause of angina pectoris and sudden death in many patients.

While Jenner withheld publishing his findings, he did write to Dr. Heberden, who was the accepted authority on the disease, angina pectoris. In the letter, Jenner wrote about the hardening of the arteries in detail, "As the heart, I believe, in every subject that has died of the angina pectoris, has been extremely loaded with fat; and as these vessels lie quite concealed in that substance, is it possible this appearance has been overlooked? The importance of the coronary arteries and how much the heart must suffer from their not being able duly to perform their functions (we should not be surprised by the painful spasms) is a subject I need not enlarge upon, therefore I shall only just remark that it is possible that the symptoms (angina pectoris and sudden death) may arise from this one circumstance."

After an argument with a colleague, Hunter complained of chest pain and suddenly expired. Since Hunter was known for his bouts of extreme temper, the manner in which he died was no surprise to Jenner. Still, Jenner went into a state of severe depression, on hearing of Hunter's death. Jenner had lost his closest friend and companion.

John Hunter, like many doctors before and after him, experimented on himself and, as a result, was responsible for his own death. Many years before his first episode of angina pectoris, he had injected himself with the venereal discharge from a patient, in order to discover if gonorrhea and syphilis were two separate diseases or nothing other than separate symptoms of one and the same disease. As a result of bad luck, the patient from whom he obtained the venereal discharge with which he injected himself was suffering from both gonorrhea and syphilis, and as a result, he contracted both diseases simultaneously. Not only was this mistake responsible for his coming to a wrong conclusion that there was a single venereal disease, and not two, but it led to his developing syphilitic thickening of the coronary arteries which was finally what caused his death.

Hunter, during his lifetime, was known as an investigator whose powers of observation were magnificent but, like Leonardo da Vinci, he was disadvantaged by his lack of literary coherence. He was quick to recognize analogies, had astute scientific judgment, and was unsparing of himself in the pursuit of truth, to the extent that he was, sadly, a martyr in his death. His human failing was, like many other scientists and politicians, that his writings were incoherent and written in a clumsy and poorly arranged manner.

On the other hand, the organization of his museum of Natural History influenced the formation of such museums in most of the other civilized countries.

He was a brilliant surgeon and comparative anatomist, who inspired a whole generation of young doctors who came after him. It was no accident that Hunter changed surgery from a trade to a science, and for many decades the surgeons, and not the physicians, would dominate the medical world. Surgery, after Hunter, would no longer be frequented by men of doubtful ability and reputation; he left it as an honorable branch of the healing arts.

All this was achieved in a short period of time by a man who took no pleasure in academic studies as a child, and on his deathbed he was known to whisper to a friend, "You will not easily find another John Hunter."

In the years following the death of John Hunter, Jenner had other misfortunes to overcome. First, he received word that his nephew, Stephen, had been lost at sea. The young soldier drowned on his way to the Peninsular War when the troopship he was on foundered off the coast of Dorset, the southernmost part of England, a disreputable area known for its looting of wrecked ships. Another nephew, George, who was his assistant and constant companion, decided to leave his apprenticeship and go to Newfoundland to work with the medical missionary and family friend, the Reverend John Clinch. It was the same Reverend Clinch to whom Jenner wrote, after Catharine gave birth to their first child, Edward.

But above all, the greatest calamity occurred when the Jenner family was exposed to an epidemic of typhus. Catharine and his children remained well but Jenner's brother, the Reverend Henry Jenner, died of the disease, and Jenner himself scarcely survived a bout of typhus.

Epidemic typhus, more commonly known as typhus fever, is caused by an organism that is extremely small, smaller than a bacteria and only a little larger than a virus. It was this vicious little organism that nearly cost Jenner his life, and while he survived, he was extremely ill, and had a prolonged and difficult convalescence. The organism which causes the disease is most frequently spread by the body louse. Typhus fever has plagued human beings for well over 2000 years and is known to have decimated the population of Athens in 430 B.C. During the many early European wars, louse-infected soldiers were a major source of spreading the disease. In Jenner's case, however, he probably was exposed to body lice, when he remained overnight caring for one of his patients who lived on a run-down farm in the country.

During his illness, Jenner's many doctor friends, who were concerned for his survival, were constantly visiting him and offering suggestions. Unfortunately, there was no specific treatment for the disease. Survival depended upon a strong physical constitution, good nursing care, and a substantial portion of luck.

15

THE PROF WAS MORE DETERMINED than ever to talk about Jenner's discovery of vaccination. Deviating from this topic of the discussion was taking more time than he planned. Always determined to complete what he had started, the Prof attempted to direct the conversation back to Jenner.

"It is time that we examine just how Jenner made his great discovery."

While the Prof's tone of voice made his proposal sound like a suggestion, everyone knew that it was an order, so no one objected. The hour was late and they, too, were anxious to complete the discussion in the shortest time possible, so that they could get to bed, for they knew that the children would be up early and anxious to continue exploring the old house.

In order to move things along, the Prof started the discussion, "You must remember that, as part of many scientific discoveries, luck plays a major role, not once but twice. First, through luck, an individual has an unplanned meeting with an unexpected natural event; second, the observer of the naturally occurring event must be inquisitive enough to search for a rational explanation for what has happened. Luck was with Jenner, the day that the dairymaid told him that she could not contract smallpox, because she had already had cowpox. Fortunately, Jenner had the fertile, inquisitive mind needed to investigate this phenomenon. Serendipity, the gift of finding something good accidentally, has been important in many major scientific discoveries. The word was coined by Horace Walpole in 1754 and was taken from *The Three Princes of Serendip,* a fairy tale in which the princes make such unexpected discoveries.

Cedric, never one to miss an opportunity to be critical or sarcastic, commented, "There are those who have suggested that it took Jenner an inordinate amount of time to develop and prove the usefulness of his discovery, while others have accused him of being awkward and dilatory."

The Prof was quick to take up the gauntlet. "Cedric, let's try to be somewhat more charitable. It is helpful to remember that eighteenth century science, in general, advanced at a slow pace—at times an extremely slow pace, by our standards. Large scientific laboratories financed by princely government grants did not exist, as they do today. It was quite the opposite; a scientist usually worked alone, or occasionally with an assistant, at a laboratory in his home, and he used his own money to support his research."

Murray, too, was offended by Cedric's remarks, "We must not forget that Jenner was a country doctor, always at the beck and call of his patients, most of whom lived in the country a considerable distance away. Remember too, Cedric, that distance in those days was a measure of how fast a horse could travel, and time, for most country people, was gauged by sunrise and sunset."

Impatient to enter the discussion, Sarah said, "For a man of Jenner's social status, custom dictated how much of his time was spent dressing or even eating. Grooming was a time-consuming ritual for a gentleman, and the main meal of the day, with all its social amenities, could last for hours."

Prof always eager to push the conversation forward, continued, "Jenner, by nature, was observant and inquisitive, and under Dr. Hunter's tutelage he improved these natural abilities. All his life, Jenner followed Hunter's dictum to him, 'don't think about it; do the experiment.'

"While Hunter understood Jenner's undue interest in cowpox, he did not support his ideas, since he viewed the study of cowpox as an obstacle to their cooperative comparative anatomy studies which, of course, were Hunter's primary interest.

"From the beginning, Jenner saw what others before him had failed to see, namely that cowpox had the potential of being a safe way of protecting people against smallpox. He was self-confident and persistent about exploring the potential value of cowpox. But there was more to it than that. He seemed to be a man on a crusade, hoping to do the work that God set out for him, protecting his fellowman from the terrible disease, smallpox.

"Remember, things weren't easy for him; he faced disbelief and scorn for his radical ideas. That a cow disease, cowpox, could protect a person from contracting a disease, smallpox, known only to humans, was an idea that the local doctors, and even most of his friends, considered silly, nothing more than 'an old wive's tale.'"

Jimmy had a feeling of deep respect for Jenner and he came to his defense. "There have always been people, such as Cedric, who have categorized Jenner, more or less, as a bumbling, lazy country doctor who, one day, stumbled on an idea that cowpox could prevent smallpox. Supposedly, he then wrote a story about it and, afterwards, went back to doctoring poor farmers and their families.

"Maybe, if we can clarify the obstacles that Jenner had to overcome in order to prove the merits of cowpox, then, perhaps, Cedric will be more respectful of him."

"Fine, Jimmy." the Prof said.

Immediately, Ruth Goldman said, "Prof, I think that we should say something with reference to how people regarded smallpox, in the eighteenth century, at the time Jenner began his study of cowpox. His vaccination discovery was a quantum leap in our knowledge about the transmission and prevention of what is known by us to be a viral disease."

The Prof reluctantly agreed, for to do otherwise would have been to no avail; when Ruth decided on a course of action, no one could prevail against her. Besides, the Prof did not want to appear rude by denying her request, though his goal now was to prevent prolonging the discussion. "Yes, Ruth, it would be useful, and suppose you lead the discussion, since it is something that you are familiar with."

"By the eighteen century, smallpox had replaced plague as the worst disease in Europe," Ruth said, "and outbreaks of smallpox occurred in all the major cities of Europe. London alone experienced five epidemics in a period of three decades, 1719 to 1749. Things had gotten so bad, that during the second half of the century, in Europe alone, 400,000 people a year died of smallpox, and it was responsible for a third of all the cases of blindness.

"There was a sense of futility among the populace on account of the disease being both incomprehensible and untreatable. The people had a right to be frightened. They couldn't see or understand the mysterious forces that were attacking them, but they did understand that, once they contracted the disease, there was no useful treatment. Under these circumstances, the people turned to their gods and goddesses for help and protection. For example, in China, Buddhists, Taoists and Confucians honored their own special smallpox goddess, hoping that, in some way, they would be protected.

"In India, since smallpox existed there for over three thousand years, the disease became interlaced with their day-to-day living. In the northern part of India, the goddess of smallpox was known as Shitala Mata. Worshipping Shitala has taken place for nearly a thousand years. Shrines have been erected to her, at which the people pray for her help, while others keep images of her in their homes. A festival honoring Shitala occurs in March during the hot, dry season, when smallpox frequently occurs. Like most such deities, Shitala possessed the power to impose the disease or to cure or prevent it.

"Myths abound about Shitala, who is depicted as a wide-eyed goddess, traveling on the back of a lactating female donkey, and carrying a broom and water pot. She is married to Shiva the Destroyer and does her damage by spreading poisonous grains that cause the pustules of smallpox.

"Tradition has it that if Shitala Mata, also known as a 'cooling mother,' accepts the peasant offerings and is cooled with aromatic baths, she will withhold her wrath; if not, she will impose the punishment of fever and rash of the dreaded smallpox. All sorts of methods were used to please the goddess. For example, to keep her from infecting their children, village women placed jugs of cool water and bowls of delicious food on their roofs, as a way of appeasing the goddess. It was unfortunate that such folklore prevented real protection when vaccination became available in India, since some of the worshippers of Shitala withheld vaccinating their children for fear of invoking her wrath. Because the village people were dealing with an unknown quantity, they imputed the cause of smallpox to many things, such as, angry gods, noxious gases or an imbalances of the body humors.

"Jenner called the mysterious substance that caused smallpox a virus, a Latin word meaning 'a poisonous force.' Of course, it was a quite different interpretation of the word, virus, than is used today. The confusing thing is that smallpox is, in modern terms, a viral disease. The word, virus, refers to a living ultramicroscopic organism that consists of nucleic acid, RNA or DNA, encased in a protein, which reproduces only within living cells."

Murray continued with the Jenner story.

"After returning to Berkeley...."

◆   ◆   ◆

After returning to Berkeley, Jenner spent the next six years catering to the needs of his patients, and did no research to advance his interest in cowpox.

Besides his medical skills, his abilities as a surgeon were frequently needed throughout the county of Gloucestershire.

While still single and in his early twenties, Jenner was leading a full and active life, in addition to fulfilling requests from Hunter for animal and biological samples for his museum.

Still, during these early years in practice, he frequently recalled the dairymaid's disquieting remark about how having had cowpox prevented her from contracting smallpox. While he continued to use variolation as a form of smallpox prevention, he did so without zeal, for he always felt that there had to be a better way of preventing the disease.

In truth, during his first six years in Berkeley, there was little opportunity for Jenner to do research on smallpox, because the disease came in cycles and had been absent from the county most of the time. Cowpox presented the same problem; it wasn't always present in the farming communities of Gloucestershire. In fact, the disease wasn't even known in most of the farming communities of England. Indeed, cowpox wasn't present in most of Europe, except for isolated areas. There were some small farming areas in Italy, where cowpox was occasionally present, and cowpox was unheard of in the American colonies, which initially made these colonies totally dependent upon Jenner for supplying them with cowpox vaccine, after he published his findings, in 1798.

When a new epidemic of smallpox presented itself, in 1778, in Gloucestershire county, including Berkeley and the surrounding farming areas, Jenner was ready. Because of the epidemic, Jenner was kept busy variolating those individuals who had never had the disease. Variolation or smallpox inoculation, as Lady Montagu called it, was still being used in England. It was during the time that Jenner was performing this procedure, throughout the farming communities, that he concluded there was more to the dairymaid's cowpox story than that it was just an "old wive's tale," as many would have him believe. Jenner best relates what happened in one of his publications.

He says, "My attention to this singular disease was first excited by observing, that among those whom in the country (farming community) I was frequently called upon to inoculate (with smallpox), many resisted every effort to give them the smallpox. These patients I found had (previously) undergone a disease they called the cow-pox, contracted by milking cows affected with a peculiar eruption on their teats."

What Jenner learned by talking to the farmers was that the older generation of farmers were only vaguely familiar with the idea that having the cowpox prevented an individual from contracting smallpox, even though the knowledge had been available for a very long time. He also noted that very few farmers and dairymaids, who had contracted cowpox, realized that they were immune to smallpox, because variolation was rarely performed on them until recently, when the procedure was made more acceptable.

For example, it was when Jenner tried to give the people in the farming community a mild case of smallpox, by variolation, and many of them did not react to the smallpox injection, because they were already immune to the disease, did they realize that their immunity was due to the fact that they previously had contracted cowpox.

Pox houses or inoculation hospitals were used for variolation. Patients were expected to undergo fasting, bleeding and purging, prior to being inoculated with smallpox. Charges for these services were expensive so that only those with adequate funds could afford to pay the fees. Daniel Sutton, in 1760, did away with the preparation, used a smaller incision and less of the inoculum which produced a milder form of smallpox and decreased the risk of death.

Despite the negative reaction of most doctors to the use of cowpox for preventing smallpox, Jenner could not be deterred from pursuing his research. It was during these years that he invariably harangued his medical colleagues and friends about the virtues of cowpox. Finally, he was shunned by most of his old companions and friends. Jenner by nature was sensitive to rebuke and criticism, but their negative remarks about cowpox failed to weaken his enthusiasm.

More and more, during the 1778 epidemic, Jenner came to realize that what he was preaching about cowpox was true, and he was now in relentless search of corroborative evidence.

Still, there were legitimate arguments against cowpox. There were those who claimed that there were many individuals who previously had had the cowpox infection and subsequently developed smallpox. Jenner concluded, correctly, that there had to be different types of lesions on the cows' utters, which were transmitted to the hands of the milkers, that were not true cowpox, and, therefore, could not protect against smallpox. Upon investigating, he established that both farmers and doctors referred to any lesion on a cow's utter as cowpox. Jenner realized that the lack of differentiation of the lesions on the cows' utters was befuddling, and that not all lesions offered protection against smallpox. Clearly then, he must first identify which lesion caused cowpox and was capable of protecting an individual against smallpox.

At this critical juncture in his research, Jenner let it be known to the farming community that he wanted to examine all lesions on the udders of cows. Fortunately, the farmers cooperated with his request, notifying him whenever they had an infected cow, and no matter the distance he had to travel, Jenner examined each infected cow. He determined that most of the lesions that he was called to see were either simple mastitis or abrasions, but, with each visit, Jenner learned how to classify each of the various lesions that occur on the cows' udders. Prior to Jenner's investigation, these lesions were all given the generic name of cowpox. At last, he was able to identify which of the lesions were true cowpox and capable of preventing smallpox. These lesions he named "true cowpox" and all the other lesions were named "spurious cowpox" meaning false cowpox.

The more Jenner learned about the true cowpox lesions, the greater was his confidence that cowpox was able to prevent smallpox, as the dairymaids had claimed. This time, however, he refrained from telling his medical colleagues and friends what he had accomplished; instead he elected to keep his own counsel, with the one exception being his friend, Gardner. Gardner, the literary man and poet, was the person who continually offered him support and understanding, during his long and laborious research.

Jenner enjoyed telling his friend the tale of the resourceful mother and the cooperative cow. When the mother learned of the special lesions on the udders of cows that prevented smallpox, being a poor woman she decided on an inexpensive method of preventing her five children from contracting the disease. She had a cow with the cowpox lesions on its udders, so she encouraged the children to play with the cow's udders; eventually, all the children developed cowpox lesions on their hands and, in effect, had thereby vaccinated themselves against smallpox.

At the same time that he solved the mystery of the true cowpox lesion, Jenner was presented with a new dilemma. He was called to a farm to care for a field-hand who had been caring for a horse with a diseased heel. The disease, unique to horses, was called grease. The man had treated the horse's heel and, immediately afterwards, milked one of the cows on the farm. Sometime later, both the field-hand and the cow developed the classical lesions of cowpox.

Subsequently, he observed a similar case where a male servant attended a horse with grease and was, shortly thereafter, sent to another farm to milk the cows. Later, both the servant and the cows developed typical cowpox lesions. In order to explain what had happened, Jenner assumed that the disease, grease, in the horse, was the source of the cowpox lesions in both the servant and the cows.

From these experiences, Jenner would later write that grease in the horse and cowpox in the cow and man were all variant forms of cowpox in animals and in man. It was an assumption that he could never prove, and later when published, he was censured by his opponents for this theory.

As was usual, the cowpox epidemic lasted only a limited time in the dairy district of Gloucestershire, but, before it ended, Jenner was certain that he could identify the true lesions of cowpox on the udders of cows or on the hands of the dairymaids. To further verify his findings and aid others, Jenner had an artist, Mr. Cuff, make drawings of the lesions of true and spurious cowpox to demonstrate these differences.

When Jenner wrote his thesis on cowpox inoculation, which would later be known as vaccination, as a means of preventing smallpox, he gave a detailed description of a cowpox vesicle on the udder of a cow and hand of a dairymaid. He wrote that, "The lesions first appear as 'pale blue colour' vesicles, surrounded by an inflammatory area of red discoloration, which later progress to irregular pustules. The animals appear sick and the milk production is decreased. It is at this time that lesions of the same type appear on the hands and wrists of the person milking the cow. The lesions on the hands quickly begin to suppurate or discharge pus. The individual now begins to develop signs of a generalize infection, feeling tired and weary, with pains in the muscles and joints. The person remains ill for from one to four days, after which there is complete recovery, except for ulcerated lesions remaining at the site of the original sores."

To top off his latest observations, he finally disclosed to his medical colleagues his finding of what was a true cowpox lesion on the udder of a cow. To his dismay, they still refused to believe him, claiming they had seen too many patients with smallpox, after previously having had typical cowpox lesions.

Even though Jenner had examined the cows and identified the lesions that he knew were responsible for producing cowpox lesions on the hands of the milkers, and they had not, he still could not dismiss their negative remarks without further sturdy.

16

THE PROF WAS PLEASED the discussion was now headed in the right direction. "Very good, Murray." Then, turning to the other guests, he said, "I think that it is now clearer that Jenner didn't discover the importance of cowpox simply by having some dairymaid tell him a tale about it, as some people would have us believe. There was much hard work and good scientific thinking that went into it, as Murray has just now told us."

Valerie interrupted, "Prof, please bear with me. Since I'm not a medical person, I want to make sure that I understood Murray's presentation about the problems Jenner had to struggle with, in proving the benefits of cowpox."

The Prof agonized over the options of being a gentleman, or being rude and denying Valerie an opportunity to speak. He chose the former. "Yes, Valerie, by all means, tell us what you got out of Murray's remarks."

"Well, we learned that Jenner was still apprenticed to Mr. Ludlow, in the 1760's, when a dairymaid told him that she could not contract smallpox, because she previously had the cowpox. This was the first time that he had heard this claim. It seems to me that it was not until 1778, which was eighteen years later, when Jenner was back in Berkeley and a major smallpox epidemic took place in Gloucestershire, that his interest in the subject was again stimulated. It was during this new epidemic, when Jenner attempted to variolate people on the farms, that some of them failed to react to the smallpox inoculation, since they previously had cowpox. It was at this point that Jenner decided there may be something to the dairymaid's story. I'm trying to simplify this complex matter. You don't mind, do you, Prof?"

The Prof shook his head to indicate "no" and gestured with his hand for her to continue. Valerie carried on with her summation.

"Jenner now faced a real predicament. There were many individuals who were known to have had the cowpox disease and still contracted smallpox, sometime later in their lives. And I think it is here that we see the brilliance of Jenner's mind coming to a quick and correct decision. He reasoned that there must be many different kinds of lesions on the udders of cows, and most of them were not related to the cowpox lesion that prevented smallpox.

"He then was able to identify only one lesion as true cowpox, and all the others as spurious or fake cowpox, which did not prevent smallpox.

"Excuse me, Prof, if I am reverting to layman's language instead of using the correct medical terms."

The Prof smiled and said, "You're doing just fine, continue."

Valerie sat back in her chair and said, "Well, that seems to be where Murray left off, Prof."

Cedric, always quick to express an opinion, remarked, "Very nice, Valerie, but it was an oversimplification of what really happened. Besides there were people who were critical of the scientific value of some of his studies."

This time, Sarah, his wife, came to Valerie's rescue. "Please, Cedric, Valerie's commentary was only a summary and not a scientific critique of Jenner's work. And it was a good summary which brought us up-to-date on the early part of his discovery."

Cedric never one to take criticism easily, responded, "Jenner had his critics, many of them, and I don't think that we should gloss over this."

Sarah, visibly annoyed with her husband, quickly replied, "Give it up, Cedric. Put it to rest."

The Prof realized that the amount of time they had spent on the topic was causing people to become a little testy, so he decided to act as the arbitrator and calm everyone's nerves. "Of course you are right, Cedric, and we still have adequate time to mention the many controversies surrounding Jenner. However, much of this faultfinding was not of his making. But in all fairness, when we get to these difficulties, I will ask you to present your side of the story.

Prof then looked over at Sarah and said, "Thank you for your help."

During the verbal give and take, Iris sat quietly in her overstuffed chair, close to the now useless fire. Nevertheless, she was not to be denied and decided to speak up. "There was a lot going on at the same time that Jenner was studying cowpox. Variolation was still being extensively used in England and throughout Europe, in spite of the fact that the doctors now saw it as a procedure that could prove to be hazardous to the individual and the community. Some argued that it wasn't logical for the doctors to make people sick, in order to keep them from harm. Some clergymen claimed variolation was evil and it was in opposition to God's divine plan. The argument about the virtues and evils of variolation continued to be debated throughout the eighteenth century, ever since Lady Montagu introduced the practice into England, early in the century.

"By the last part of the eighteenth century, many European countries had banned the practice of variolation, for fear of it being a source of starting a new smallpox epidemic.

"In England the practice began losing favor in 1783, when King George III's son died, as a consequence of being variolated. In addition, smallpox pus was also found to be a way of spreading other diseases to the person being variolated. Diseases, such as tuberculosis and syphilis were the two most common. The main objection to variolation was that, while the person being inoculated with the smallpox matter may become only moderately ill, he was still able to spread the disease to other individuals, which could be the source of a new smallpox epidemic."

"Thank you, Iris," the Prof mumbled, for he, too, was showing signs of tiring and perhaps becoming a bit surly.

But the Prof was not one to acquiesce, and like Jenner, he was steadfast. "Jimmy, would you mind continuing the story where Murray left off?"

"Okay, Prof. I'll do my best. By 1782...."

◆   ◆   ◆

By 1782, the epidemic of cowpox was over. There were no more cowpox lesions on the cows' udders to be studied. Jenner was disappointed and discouraged. Later, after he and Catharine were married, it was she who comforted and encouraged him, during his periods of depression, to continue his research.

When his oldest son, Edward, was born there was still no cowpox among the herds of the farming community. Jenner had hoped to inoculate the child with cowpox but, because there was none available, he inoculated the boy with the infectious material, grease, which he obtained from the hoof of an infected horse. However, the boy did not react to the inoculation, so the outcome of this experiment proved nothing.

Another nine years would go by before a cowpox epidemic would once again return to the farms of Gloucestershire, allowing Jenner to resume his cowpox research. Meanwhile, another obstacle that he had not anticipated confronted him; namely, there were individuals who previously had cowpox and contracted smallpox, when exposed to it at a later date, indicating that they had failed to develop immunity.

Jenner concluded that, like smallpox, the contents of the cowpox lesions varied in potency, depending upon the time that the milkers were exposed to the lesions on the cows' udders. Undoubtedly, there was a critical period of time when the matter in the lesion was of maximum potency and infectivity. If the cowpox matter were removed at any other time it would fail to immunize an individual against smallpox. This assumption turned out to be correct, and from this time on, Jenner was able to extract virulent or active viral material with which to vaccinate his patients against contracting smallpox.

As added proof of the virtue of having had cowpox, Jenner began recording histories of farm individuals who, in the past, had contracted cowpox in the normal way, and were shown to be immune to smallpox after having been exposed to it naturally. After first having had cowpox, most of these individuals took care of friends or relatives with smallpox, without themselves contracting the disease. Jenner was impressed that these immune individuals had their cowpox infections many years before their exposure to smallpox, and they still remained immune to the disease. Jenner concluded that cowpox infection conferred lifetime immunity to smallpox. It was a conclusion that was not correct; the immunity lasts ten or more years but not a lifetime.

Jenner's golden opportunity, to conclusively prove his theory that cowpox immunized an individual against smallpox, presented itself in May of 1796, when a dairymaid by the name of Sarah Nelmes scratched her finger on a thorn prior to milking an infected cow. Within days the injured finger developed a typical cowpox lesion, and, thereafter, the girl was feverish, associated with feelings of physical discomfort, and soon she was unable to do her work. Finally, the illness subsided and the lesion on her finger continued to heal. Jenner knew that Sarah was exactly the patient that he was waiting for, to continue with his experiment.

After first having obtained permission from the parents to vaccinate their eight-year-old son, James Phipps, Jenner made two small scratches on the boy's arm and into them he inoculated cowpox matter taken from the finger of Sarah Nelmes.

The boy returned home with his parents, and was visited daily by Jenner, who monitored his well-being during the course of the disease. It wasn't until the seventh day that James felt discomfort and developed a tender swelling in his armpit. Two days later, there was generalized malaise, fever, loss of appetite and a desire to remain in bed. Naturally, his parents were apprehensive, but Jenner reassured them that the boy was experiencing the usual symptoms of cowpox disease, and there was nothing to worry about. To everyone's delight, the following day, James Phipps was free of his symptoms and in good health.

After another few days, the lesions on his arm crusted, and afterwards, when the crusts fell off, a small scar remained.

Four weeks later, Jenner made small incisions on both his arms, barely breaking the skin, and inoculated the incisions with smallpox matter. He performed what was a typical variolation procedure being used at that time. The boy failed to react to the smallpox injections, indicating that he was immune to the disease.

Finally, after a few months, Jenner repeated the smallpox inoculation. Again, James failed to react to the variolation, confirming that he was indeed immune to smallpox.

The Phipps experiment established Jenner's contention that vaccination was a valid and safe way to prevent smallpox. He vowed that, "I shall now pursue my experiments with redoubled ardour." Unfortunately, it was a promise that he could not carry out for another two years, because it took that long for cowpox to once again infect the cow herds of Gloucestershire.

James Phipps' vaccination was a seminal event in the history of smallpox, and July 1796 was to be known as "the year of discovery." Jenner's premise about the protective value of cowpox was validated. Unfortunately though, the discovery had gone unnoticed, except for a few of Jenner's friends and the residents of Cheltenham, where Jenner usually spent his summers in a rented house on Main Street. Later he bought a house there.

News of the Phipps experiment reached some of the doctors in London, whose profitable medical practices depended upon the variolation of their patients. The response from these doctors was an immediate rejection of Jenner and his discovery.

After a memorable summer in Cheltenham, Jenner and his family returned to Berkeley for the winter. Before long, Catharine and the children left Berkeley and returned to Cheltenham, because of the severity of the winter of 1796–1797. Jenner remained in Berkeley and eventually went to live at Berkeley Castle to care for Lady Berkeley, who, after giving birth, had a life threatening postnatal reaction.

Lord Berkeley's peccadillos were well known throughout the country and his moral behavior was not above reproach. It seems that Lady Berkeley, previously known as Mary Cole, had come to the Castle as a domestic servant and had cohabited with Lord Berkeley for eleven years, before they married. Their marriage resulted in many births; however, an illegitimate son was known to have been born before the marriage took place. Jenner presided over all of Lady Berkeley's deliveries, and was privy to all that was taking place at the Castle. While Lord Berkeley was known as a notorious libertine, whatever took place at the Castle was held in strictest confidence by Jenner.

Since 1789, Jenner had been a respected member of the Royal Society, where he had been recommended for membership by his mentor, Dr. John Hunter. Jenner's election into the Royal Society was not for his work in medicine, but for his contributions to natural history. His studies on the nesting habits of the cuckoo bird were paramount in his being appointed to membership.

Jenner, therefore, decided to write a short summary of his research with cowpox, which eventually led to the discovery of vaccination. The centerpiece of his paper was the vaccination of James Phipps, which resulted in James' immunity to smallpox. Jenner was a member of the Royal Society; he knew Sir Joseph Banks, the president of the Society since 1787; he corresponded with Banks for years; and supplied him with fauna specimens from West of England. For all these reasons, Jenner expected a favorable reception for his cowpox paper, when he submitted it, but that did not happen.

In 1796, Jenner's cowpox paper was carefully read by Banks and a few other members of the Society, and returned to Jenner after being rejected. The short paper described but one experiment and Jenner's varied arguments supporting his contention that having had cowpox protected an individual from contracting smallpox.

Along with the rejected paper, Banks wrote Jenner a short note to the effect that the paper lacked adequate scientific proof to support his far-reaching conclusion about cowpox. Included in the note was the advice that, if the paper were read before the Society, it would damage Jenner's well earned scientific reputation, a reputation which he so rightly deserved for his work about the cuckoo bird's unusual behavior.

In retrospect, some have questioned Bank's rejection of the cowpox paper as a malicious act against Jenner, a conclusion which does not seem justified, based upon Jenner's behavior after receiving the rejection. It is more likely that Banks, the perpetual pedantic, would not or could not accept that Jenner, an unknown country doctor, was capable of proving such a daring conclusion. Jenner decided to carry on with his research and ignore the rejection of his initial studies of cowpox and vaccination.

But it was not until early in 1798 that Jenner had the opportunity to continue with his experiments. This time he was to inoculate two young boys. One boy was inoculated with matter taken from the hand of a man infected with the disease, grease, which originated from the hoof of a horse that he was treating. The other boy was inoculated with cowpox matter taken directly from the udder of an infected cow. It was important for him to use young children for his vaccination studies, since it was the only way that he could be certain that they had never been exposed to either cowpox or smallpox.

During these inoculations, an unfortunate thing happened. The first boy who received the disease, grease, contracted a secondary disease, unrelated to the inoculation, and died. The second boy, William Summers, who received the cowpox vaccination, developed typical cowpox symptoms and recovered after four days.

At this point, Jenner designed a series of experiments to prove that cowpox could be maintained by serial transmission in humans. With cowpox matter taken from William Summer's lesion, Jenner vaccinated a man named William Pead. With cowpox matter taken from Pead's lesions, he then vaccinated several other people including Hannah Excell, a seven-year-old girl. It was cowpox matter taken from Hannah's lesions with which Jenner vaccinated his younger son, Robert. Unfortunately, Robert's vaccination failed to take, but three other individuals, vaccinated at the same time, developed a positive vaccination reaction.

Finally, Jenner completed his experiments feeling that he had done enough to prove that vaccination, using cowpox matter, was sufficient to prevent these individuals from ever contracting the frightful disease, smallpox.

He stated that, "After the many fruitless attempts to give the smallpox to those who had the cowpox, it did not appear necessary, nor was it convenient to me to inoculate the whole of those who had been the subject of these late trials, though I thought it right to see the effects of variolous matter on some of them, particularly William Summers, the first of the patients who had been infected with the matter taken from the cow. He was, therefore, inoculated with variolous matter from a fresh pustule but, as in the preceding cases, his system did not feel the effects in the smallest degree."

This was a decision by Jenner which resulted in some negative consequences, and for which he would later be criticized. But what he did in no way changed the results of his experiment. In hindsight, it would have been a wiser choice for him to have performed variolation on all the individuals that he vaccinated with the cowpox that was passed on by serial transfer.

He then proceeded to accumulate additional information on individuals who had previously contracted their cowpox infections, while milking infected cows. All these individuals showed no reaction to variolation, indicating that they were immune to smallpox. Armed with the additional cases supporting his premise of the preventative value of cowpox, Jenner elected now to publish his completed work on the efficacy of vaccination as a means of preventing smallpox infection.

But before publishing his thesis this time, he had his many doctor friends critically review his work. With their encouragement, Jenner, in 1798, prepared a small pamphlet, which he published at his own expense, putting forth his findings and conclusions on vaccination.

17

IT WAS MURRAY WHO BEGAN SPEAKING, as soon as Jimmy finished his presentation. "Cedric, he said, "you have to admit that Jenner did some exceptionally fine scientific work, in order to prove that vaccination was capable of preventing smallpox, without producing illness in the person being vaccinated or causing a cowpox epidemic. Remember, there were even those who referred to Jenner's discovery as, 'Jenner's earth-shattering development.'"

"I don't know," Cedric responded, "it seems to me that it was no more than just plain good scientific research; no more than that. I must admit, though, that vaccination turned out to be a very useful medical tool."

It was obvious that Murray was visibly shaken by Cedric's insipid remark and needed a moment or two to regain his composure. Murray's physical response to Cedric's tasteless comment was more or less a combination of things. Cedric had a personality that tended to unnerve people, especially individuals of a more sensitive nature, who disliked responding acrimoniously towards others; but, the lateness of the hour was also adding to Murray's annoyance.

"Cedric," he began again, "try to remember that Jenner's work was done in the last part of the eighteenth century when research was carried on by inquisitive individuals, working at home, usually alone, and using their own money to finance their research. But, Cedric, we have already discussed that, so let's not rehash it now.

"After Jenner identified which lesion on the udders of cows were those that caused cowpox in the dairymaids, he was confronted with another dilemma. Namely, not all of the cow's true cowpox lesions that produced lesions on the hands of the dairymaids assured them of immunity against smallpox.

"Based upon his knowledge of smallpox, Jenner knew that there was a limited period of time that the disease was infective. He reasoned that the same must be true of the cowpox disease—that not all true cowpox lesions were completely infective. There had to be a limited period of time when the lymph material removed from a cowpox lesion was strong enough to produce immunity in the person being inoculated with it. And, of course, this turned out to be true.

Murray continued, "Jenner knew that he had to take his experimentation one step further, to prove his point that having had cowpox, a person was immune to the disease, smallpox. As you remember, for this experiment, Jenner inoculated (vaccinated) James Phipps with cowpox lymph that he removed from a lesion on the hand of Sarah Nelmes. Later, Phipps was proven to be immune to smallpox.

"The Phipps experiment was crucial to proving Jenner's thesis, and he was elated with the results. He depicted this epic discovery in the following manner, in a note to a close friend. "But now listen to the most delightful part of my story. The boy has since been inoculated for the Smallpox which, as I ventured to predict, produced no effects. I shall now pursue my Experiments with redoubled ardor."

"The importance of the Phipps experiment was more than just the boy's vaccination. Jenner was able to prove that an animal disease, cowpox, acquired accidentally by a person while milking an infected cow, rendered the individual immune to a human disease, smallpox; and that the cowpox lymph removed from a cowpox lesion on the hand of one person could be used successfully to vaccinate another individual against smallpox. Later, he was able to show that cowpox lymph could be passed on through many individuals—which he referred to as serially transferred—and still be capable of successfully vaccinating each individual. It may seem simple now, but in the 18th century, this was an important milestone in the history of medicine.

"Before publishing the results of the Phipps experiment, Jenner gathered additional information on a group of adults who previously had cowpox and failed to respond to his variolating them, indicating that they were immune to smallpox. He considered these data sufficient to be published and offered his paper to Sir Joseph Banks, his old friend and president of the Royal Society, who, you will recall, rejected Jenner's first paper in 1796.

"In the eighteenth century, what was different from past centuries was the notion that science had a social responsibility. Jenner understood this and acted accordingly. He was part of a century that had known three social revolutions that changed how the world performed: the Industrial Revolution in 1760; the American Revolution in 1775; and the French Revolution in 1789. To a lesser degree, during the eighteenth century, there was another revolution, a medical revolution, of which Jenner was one of its leaders.

"There are times when an ordinary man...."

◆ ◆ ◆

There are times when an ordinary man gets entangled in social or scientific change that forces him to become somebody out-of-the ordinary, or above the crowd. For Jenner, once the *Inquiry* was published, his life changed.

It has been said that no small booklet ever made the name of its author so famous; and this is probably true; but fame came neither quickly, nor without conflict.

Near the end of April 1798, with a completed manuscript of the *Inquiry* in hand, Jenner was off to London to have it printed. It was the culmination of a work that lasted many years, and contained within it his dream of doing something noble that would benefit mankind. After a long and uncomfortable coach ride to London, he arrived covered with dust and totally exhausted. Nevertheless, he was impatient to see his scientific achievement in print for all to read, for he knew he was about to receive recognition for his triumph over smallpox.

It was nearly twenty-five years since he last saw London. In spite of that, it held no charm for him, yet London was where he must be, if vaccination was to receive universal approval and replace variolation as the accepted practice for preventing smallpox.

Living in London was a luxury that he could ill afford, so he had hoped to have the *Inquiry* printed and distributed without delay. He was convinced the *Inquiry* could be commercially printed and sold without a cost to him. He was short of money, and paying the cost of printing the booklet, therefore, was a financial imposition that he had hoped to avoid. While Jenner was not poor, still his medical practice in the farming community of Berkeley provided him with only a limited income.

After many months living in London, he was unable to find a printer who would sponsor the pamphlet, so he acquiesced to having the *Inquiry* printed at his own expense.

In June of 1798, the pamphlet was published with the imposing title of: *An Inquiry into the causes and effects of The Variolae Vaccinae, a disease discovered in some of the western counties of England, particularly Gloucestershire, and known by the name of The Cow Pox.* Jenner used the Latin word vacca for cow and devised the term vaccination.

While the discovery marked a milestone in medical history, the pamphlet had a disturbing effect on its readers. To many, the contents of the pamphlet were an enigma, and its ideas were accepted by as many as rejected them.

It was a small book, a mere seventy-five pages of large type with wide margins and generous spacing. The book had to be read in the context of its time; for example, 18th century scientific literature frequently began by referring to the morality of the material that it contained, and Jenner conformed to this custom. He assumes that man has sinned by living a life of luxury and deviant behavior, and disease is the punishment for his sins. It was man's close association with certain animals that has made him vulnerable to disease; and he says that this close association was with the dog, cat, cow, hog, sheep and horse, which, for a variety of purposes, man brought under his care and dominion.

But it is in the body of the pamphlet that he proves his thesis that vaccination, which contains the disease, cowpox, is capable of protecting man against the horrible disease, smallpox; and it does this without disabling the recipient of vaccination or putting the community at risk of an epidemic of cowpox. Jenner proves this by giving a short description of cowpox and follows up with an account of twenty-eight individuals who had cowpox, sometime in their past, and later failed to develop smallpox, when exposed to it naturally, or did not respond to it when they were inoculated with smallpox. The third part of the report contains the most convincing proof for the usefulness of vaccination. In it he gives the history of the dairymaid, Sarah Nelmes, and the eight-year-old boy, James Phipps. He tells how Sarah had contracted cowpox while milking an infected cow, and afterwards developed classical cowpox lesions on her hand. Jenner removed some infectious matter and inserted it into two superficial incisions that he had made on the arm of James Phipps. Later, he inoculated the boy with smallpox matter and proved that he was immune to the disease, smallpox.

The Nelmes\Phipps experiment confirmed that the cowpox virus was transferable from the cow to man. But more importantly, the same virus could be transferred between persons by vaccination and still protect against smallpox.

His early case presentations were based upon presumptive evidence, namely case histories from the individuals with whom he spoke. The later case presentations consist of patients that he vaccinated, and confirmed his theory that cowpox infection protects against smallpox.

Next, he presents information, from his practical experience, on the procedure that was to be universally known as vaccination, and closes his pamphlet with a long discourse on his observation of cowpox and the use of vaccination.

Jenner forthrightly states that his data supports his assertion, "that the Cow-pox protects the human constitution from the infection of the Small-pox." And if this was all he had to claim, his medical research would still be acknowledged and his name revered in medicine. But there was still more to come.

He proceeded to say, that while he can not decisively prove it, because of circumstances beyond his control, namely, the disease in horses was no longer present in his area, he still believes that the disease in the horse is the cause of cowpox in the cow. Unfortunately, it is a statement that he would later retract.

The demonstration that cowpox lymph was still protective against smallpox, after having been serially passed through five different individuals, was one of his most useful experiments. Arm-to-arm serial vaccination, as the process was referred to, demonstrated that it was no longer necessary to depend upon cowpox disease in the cow herds as a reservoir of cowpox lymph for vaccination.

It was pivotal to his discovery of vaccination, when he showed that not all the lesions on the udders of cows contained the cowpox virus, and that only true cowpox lesions contained lymph capable of vaccinating against smallpox.

Notwithstanding the fact that the *Inquiry* produced some disagreements amongst the doctors, Jenner's work was valid and correct, as many of his detractors failed to realize at the time.

With great modesty and humility, Jenner concludes the *Inquiry* saying that he knows that his work is incomplete, so he will continue with his studies, but in the meantime, he prays that this work will be beneficial to all mankind. In this simple statement, he demonstrated the qualities of a great man striving to live up to the code of medicine that the patient and mankind should be the benefactors of his knowledge and training.

Jenner claimed in the *Inquiry* that vaccination produced life-long immunity against smallpox. Unfortunately it, too, was a statement that he would later have to alter. But after the *Inquiry* was printed, the statement was used to disparage Jenner's reputation and belittle his research.

During this time, however, he exhibited what, for him, was unusual behavior. He had come to London to present his foremost scientific work, and within two weeks of launching the *Inquiry*, he suddenly left to return to Cheltenham to be with his family.

Perhaps Jenner was expecting too much from the London doctors whose training was based on the medical writings of Hippocrates (460 B.C.) and Galen (130 A.D), ancient physicians who held that the body was composed of the four "humours": blood, phlegm, yellow, and black bile. Disturbances in the balance of the four humours were the origin of disease, and to remain in good health, the four humours had to remain in balance.

Fortunately, however, there were other physicians like Jenner, whose discoveries were opening new vistas and changing medicine from an ancient art into a respectable science. One such physician, also an Englishman, was William Harvey who was educated at the Grammar School at Canterbury, Caius College, Cambridge, and Padua Medical School, Italy, one of the world's oldest medical schools. In 1616, Harvey announced his remarkable discovery how the blood circulated through the human body, which had been an unsolved mystery, since the days of Hippocrates, in ancient Greece.

Jenner's discovery that infectious material from an animal, the cowpox, could be used to protect a human against an unrelated human disease, was difficult for the medical profession to accept or to totally comprehend. And it would take another eighty years before the mechanism underlying vaccination was entirely understood.

It took the brilliant French scientist, Pasteur, to demonstrate that there were microorganisms—germs—in the infectious material that caused disease. Based upon the ground-breaking work of Jenner, Pasteur would later produce his own vaccines against rabies and anthrax.

It was also, unfortunately, that eighteenth century medicine was a combination of science and sorcery. There was a plethora of medicines used to treat patients, nearly all without merit, and most were secret formulas known only to the individual physician. Surgical treatments were equally archaic. Compound fractures, where a broken bone pierced the skin, were treated by amputation of the limb to prevent an infection, which was usually fatal. Bloodletting was still the accepted treatment for fevers. Was it any wonder then, in such an inexact medical environment, that an advanced thesis, such as the *Inquiry*, was initially poorly understood and received by the London medical community.

At a later date in time, the *Inquiry* was best summarized by Sir Benjamin Richardson when he wrote, "No book so small has been talked of so much: no book read from the original so little: no book of such dimensions has made the name of the author so famous."

18

"IF WE LIMIT THE DISCUSSION," the Prof quickly interjected, "it will speed things up and, at the same time, help us to understand why many London doctors refused to accept vaccination, after reading the *Inquiry*."

Even though the group was weary, they unanimously responded that they wished to continue. The Prof, of course, was delighted; he did not want to stop before Jenner's story was completed, even if continuing meant prolonging the evening until the early hours of the morning.

The Prof continued the story, but not before he first made an observation. "There are many types of intellectual abilities," the Prof began, "for example, a first-class chess player requires supreme concentration and retention of the movements of the objects on the board before him, to overpower his opponent; while a skilled poker play relies not only on his mental abilities to determine the value of his cards, but he must also transcend the tangible, the playing cards, and enter the mysterious world of the subconscious, the mind of his opponent, to outsmart him. Jenner, on the other hand, was analytical in his reasoning. He observed what others before him had observed but had failed to comprehend. There were a few farmers and dairymaids who knew that having had cowpox could prevent contracting smallpox, but they did not know what it all meant. And there were doctors who had heard these same rumors, but they didn't believe them. Jenner, however, had heard these same rumors and decided they were important enough to be investigated.

"Jenner soon realized that what to others were 'old wives' tales' were, in reality, experiments or accidents of scientific significance designed by nature. These so-called accidents of nature occur all the time without our realizing it, of course. For an accident of nature to be of value, it must be observed, but observed by someone with an analytical mind capable of interpreting the experiment.

"Jenner saw more than cowpox protecting the dairymaids from smallpox. He deduced, if cowpox protected the dairymaids, why not make it available to everyone? And he didn't stop there, because he concluded that if everyone were immune, smallpox could be eliminated everywhere and the smallpox virus eventually would be eliminated from the planet, since the virus could only survive in human beings. Smallpox is a uniquely human disease, which has no animal host in which it can hide and survive. It can not exist without susceptible humans, except in tissue cultures in a laboratory, of course.

"In 1979, Jenner's prediction proved correct. Smallpox was declared eliminated from our planet by the World Health Organization. It was the first disease to attain such distinction; unfortunately, it did not happen in Jenner's lifetime. Jenner was able to see beyond nature's experiment with the dairymaids. He visualized a way of obtaining salvation for all mankind by the elimination of one of nature's most dreaded scourges. Throughout his writings, he used the all-inclusive word, mankind, as the final purpose of his experimental work with cowpox vaccination."

"Come, come, Prof, it wasn't all that simple, was it?" Cedric questioned.

"Of course not, Cedric, you know that. It is a frightfully long tale from Jenner to the final elimination of smallpox from our planet. There were many, many people who took part in this outstanding accomplishment, far too many for us to mention this evening. We must, however, refer to this achievement, considering that it is an indispensable part of the smallpox story. Remember that without Jenner and his discovery of vaccination there would be no story to tell."

"Oh, I don't know about that, Prof. If Jenner hadn't discovered vaccination, eventually, some other chap would have," Cedric pressed the Prof.

"Cedric, please, let's not play one of your 'what if' games tonight. The fact is that Jenner discovered and developed vaccination as the procedure by which smallpox was eliminated," the Prof retorted somewhat angrily, sounding more exhausted than irritated. He continued, "Cedric, you can be of use to us this evening. There were objections to Jenner and his ideas, shortly after the *Inquiry* was printed and circulated. I know that you are conversant with this subject, so, perhaps, you will enlighten the rest of us."

"I'd be delighted, Prof," Cedric promptly acknowledged. "No matter how noble Jenner's intentions...."

◆   ◆   ◆

No matter how noble Jenner's intentions, he was still not beyond the range of the caustic remarks and the criticisms from the London doctors. In general, they gave the *Inquiry* a negative review. But remember, many of these same doctors had a vested interest in the continuation of variolation, since the procedure produced a lucrative income for them. If they acknowledged that Jenner's vaccination was a safer and more efficient way of preventing smallpox, they would be hurting themselves. Another problem was that some doctors were poorly educated and failed to comprehend the value of vaccination, because the idea was such a new one.

These dissident doctors concluded that the quickest and, perhaps, the easiest way to stop the use of vaccination was to attack Jenner directly and destroy his reputation. "That little country doctor," was used in a disparaging manner, and was a phrase frequently heard. In truth, if Jenner had never discovered cowpox and developed the practice of vaccination, his name would still be recorded in the annals of the history of medicine and science. While it was true that Jenner was a relatively unknown country doctor, in reality, he was also an elected member of the most learned scientific society in the world, the Royal Society. Jenner being Jenner, he avoided confrontation with those who attacked him, no matter how cruel their blows. Later, though, his friends came to his defense, in order to redeem his good name.

Back in Cheltenham, Jenner suddenly became embroiled in a dispute with an unexpected adversary, a Dr. John Ingenhousz, of Austria. Ingenhousz introduced variolation to Austria, and had successfully variolated the Empress Maria Theresa against smallpox. When the *Inquiry* appeared in print, Ingenhousz was visiting in England, as a guest of a British nobleman. Ingenhousz used his celebrity status as the personal physician to the Emperor of Austria, to disparage Jenner and besmirch the practice of vaccination.

What is true today was also true in Jenner's time. If someone disagrees with a person who has made an important but controversial discovery, a celebrity frequently is used to attack the individual rather than attack the idea directly. It all seems so backwards. Why not attack the idea or discovery? While the majority of London doctors probably agreed with Ingenhousz, it is also true that a scientific fact or principle is not established by a democratic vote or majority.

Even though Ingenhousz had the temerity to denigrate Jenner's discovery, he still had no personal experience with cowpox. In England he was staying at an estate in Wiltshire, and whatever little knowledge he had about the subject of vaccination was obtained by gossip from the local doctors who assured him that cowpox was of no value in preventing smallpox.

For whatever reason, perhaps envy, Dr. Ingenhousz, who had made a particular study of smallpox, and had variolated members of the Imperial family of Vienna and Tuscany, took offense to Jenner and his work. Even though, by now, Jenner had prepared himself for just such criticism and personal attacks, he was initially somewhat overwhelmed by the prestigious Ingenhousz. Jenner recorded in his personal notes that, "The station and character of such a man as Ingenhousz was nevertheless not to be neglected."

Dr. Ingenhousz accused Jenner of dishonest conclusions in the *Inquiry*, without himself carefully investigating the outcome of vaccinations. There are different means of deceiving oneself: by a defect in one's judgment or through self-deception, either of which can happen to a person of superior intelligence; or by passing judgment without prior knowledge, which happens to be "the tool of a fool." It was difficult to know in which category the Austrian doctor belonged.

To sully a person's name is a common practice, when knowledge is absent, and it was frequently used against Jenner by his adversaries. His opponents were constantly raising arguments, unrelated to vaccination, to conceal the true issue: that cowpox was capable of protecting an individual from contracting smallpox, and that the safest way of producing smallpox immunity was by vaccination.

Ingenhousz continued his antagonism of Jenner by writing him letters. Some of the letters were respectful of Jenner, but they were written in a manner suggesting the writer to be a person vested with great authority and pomposity. In one such letter, the esteemed Dr. Ingenhousz informed Jenner that he deliberately sought information at the dairies of Wilshire, a place where cowpox was present, and confirmed that having had cowpox was useless as a way of preventing smallpox. He then verified examples of individuals who had had cowpox and were subsequently infected with smallpox. According to Ingenhousz, false promises were made in the *Inquiry* about the security offered by vaccination. With an attitude of smugness, he then chastised Jenner by saying, "all the security which you promise from (cowpox) inoculation is so neutralized by this testimony." With additional imprudence and arrogance, Ingenhousz presumed to advise Jenner to confess that he was in error, and "prevent the disappointment which must follow from ungratified expectations."

These were harsh conclusions and a severe reprimand for Jenner. Still, even after receiving such a letter, Jenner's equanimity remained. Jenner contacted a physician in Wiltshire who assured him that in Wiltshire the lesion of true cowpox had not yet been differentiated from all the other lesions occurring on the udders of cows. It was those other lesions, which Jenner labeled as "spurious" cowpox, that failed to protect individuals from contracting smallpox. Jenner had stressed this in the *Inquiry*.

Jenner's letter, replying to Ingenhousz, was temperate indeed, for Ingenhousz's mistakes were immediately obvious to Jenner. After explaining to Ingenhousz where he went wrong, Jenner then wrote that much of his data in the *Inquiry* was preliminary. He then explained, "In the publication, I have given little more than a simple detail of the facts which came under my own inspection, and to the public I stand pledged for its veracity....Should it appear in the present instance that I have been led into error, fond as I may appear of the offspring of my labours (his conclusion), I had rather strangle it at once than suffer it to exist, and do a public injury." Jenner concludes his letter by suggesting to Ingenhousz that the doubts that he offered could be settled by using scientific testing, rather than hearsay or gossip. "Therefore I conceive it would be prudent," Jenner continues, "until further inquiry has thrown every light on the subject which it is capable of receiving, that (like those who were the objects of my experiments) all should be subject to the test of variolous (smallpox inoculation) matter who have been vaccinated for cowpox."

Much can be learned about Jenner, the man, from the contents of his letter to Ingenhousz. First there is Jenner the doctor, a learned person and a teacher, who unhesitatingly and forthrightly certifies the truthfulness (veracity) of his statements in the *Inquiry*. But no matter how much he loved what he produced, which he called, "the offspring of my labours," if the conclusions were wrong, he would strangle them rather than see them do public injury.

Regrettably, Jenner's bland letters failed to stop Ingenhousz's offensive missives. For such an august and authoritative individual as Ingenhousz, saving face came before acknowledging scientific truth. It seemed that the more Jenner tried to be humble, propitiatory and placatory towards him, the more Ingenhousz answered with rudeness and imperiousness—the standard camouflage of a lazy mind.

Jenner's tolerance for the egotistic Austrian doctor was by now wearing thin, so he decided to forgo any more letter writing. This disturbing episode ended with a snippy comment Jenner made to his friend and trusted advisor, Dr. Gardner: "This very man, Ingenhousz, knows no more of the real nature of the cowpox than Master Selwyn does of Greek: yet he (Ingenhousz) is among philosophers what (Samuel) Johnson was among the literati, and by the way, not unlike him in figure (girth). Tis no use to shoot straws at an eagle."

Ignoring Ingenhousz failed to solve Jenner's problems, since criticisms of the *Inquiry* continued to increase. As the faultfinding by Ingenhousz and others continued, Jenner again wrote to his friend Gardner, "I am beset with snarling fellows, so ignorant that they know no more of the disease they write about than the animals which generate it."

Fortunately for Jenner though, the majority of the negative reports were of a nature that he had anticipated would occur. Those who claimed that cowpox failed to prevent naturally occurring smallpox, used the spurious form of cowpox lymph, and not the true cowpox lymph that he had worked so long and hard to identify.

There were, however, two criticisms of his work that were more troublesome to dismiss, namely, that cowpox produced life-long immunity, and the source of the virus, cowpox, was the disease, grease, which originated as an infection in the heel of the horse.

Jenner knew that more research had to be done on the question of life-long immunity and that the *Inquiry* was but a provisional summary of the virtues of cowpox. The *Inquiry*, however, except for minor deficiencies, was accurate and correct, and by any standard, reflected an excellent and important piece of research that would save millions upon millions of lives.

Grease was another matter though. Jenner was tentative, when he assumed a cause-and-effect relationship between the disease, grease, in the horse and cowpox in the cow. Under pressure from continual carping, he seemed to have changed his belief that grease was the source of cowpox in the cow.

When criticisms of the *Inquiry* were at their zenith and attacks on Jenner's personal integrity and honor were continuous, the tide of battle took a sudden and complete turn, favoring Jenner. Studies, verifying his work that cowpox prevented smallpox, began being reported not only from England but from most of the European countries.

There were others who complained it took too long for him to complete his research, but these same people would also complain had his work been completed in a lesser amount of time but not nearly so carefully done. Jenner rightly concluded, "Since I can't please everyone, it is best that I please myself."

People did not understand that Jenner had responsibilities to care for his patients in both Berkeley and Cheltenham, besides looking after his family and an ailing wife, while at the same time conducting his research on cowpox vaccine. Jenner was not a rich man so the cost of his research, in both time and money, came from his medical practice. But now that his research was finished, he was ready to show the world how smallpox could be prevented, without danger to the person being vaccinated or the fear of spreading smallpox.

Jenner was happy to admit he had had help in his conquest of smallpox, for God was at his side from the beginning, guiding him and reinforcing his resolve when things were difficult. Nevertheless, he pondered, when the time came to receive honors for his achievement, how to share his tangible laurels with an intangible God.

Jenner wondered whether or not it was unfair to compare his medical achievement to that of a musical creation by a musical genius. His opus, the conquest of smallpox, was equal to any of the great musical compositions, except that his creation would save the lives of millions of people now living, as well as those not yet born. Still, Jenner reasoned that without music, man would be less than human; therefore, both great music and great medical discoveries were of equal importance.

At the very peak of the negative battle taking place around him, and at a time when he was about to be overcome by his enemies, Jenner received a letter from a simple country doctor like himself, which read:

> "My dear Sir,
>
> The cow-pox experiment has succeeded admirably. The child sickened on the seventh day, and the fever, which was moderate, subsided on the eleventh. The inflammation arising from the insertion of the virus extended to about four inches in diameter and then gradually subsided, without having been attended with pain or other inconvenience. There were no eruptions.
>
> Doctor Lister, who was formerly physician to the smallpox hospital, attended the child with me and he is convinced that it is not possible to give him the smallpox. I think the substituting of the cowpox poison for the smallpox promises to be one of the greatest improvements that has ever been made in medicine, and the more I think on the subject the more I am impressed with its importance,
>
> With great esteem,
> I am etc.
>
> Henry Cline.
>
> Lincoln's Inn Fields.
> August 9th 1798."

19

"PERHAPS, IF WE EXAMINE WHAT WE now know about smallpox and compare it with what was known about the disease in Jenner's time, we will appreciate how little real scientific information Jenner had when he made his memorable discovery," the Prof said, hoping to move the group quickly onto the next topic for discussion. "Jimmy, how about giving us some information on the smallpox virus, based upon modern virology."

"That's a tall order, Prof. Suppose I give you some simple factual information, just enough to get us by for the present," Jimmy responded. "It is essential to know that smallpox is solely a human disease and there are no animals or birds that host this virus. In other words, humans pass it to other humans. The disease, smallpox, has been eliminated in humans, even though the virus is still being grown in culture, in some laboratories. Jenner predicted that vaccination would one day free mankind of this terrible disease, and this is exactly what happened.

"There are not many viral diseases that have this unique feature of man being the only host for the virus. There are a few; chickenpox is one of them, even though the name is a misnomer.

"The virus that causes smallpox is properly named variola virus, and it is one of a large group of viruses known as true pox viruses. The cowpox virus, which we have been discussing, belongs to the same group of true pox viruses, but the host for this virus is a rodent and rarely, as we have learned, does it infect cows. Actually, there are many animals and rodents that get pox lesions, and in each animal the disease is caused by a special pox virus. For example, there are different pox viruses that cause mousepox, rabbitpox, camelpox, monkeypox, raccoonpox and more. What is of interest, though, is that vaccination not only protects against smallpox, but it also protects against some of these other animal and rodent pox diseases."

At this point Sarah, usually reticent and disinclined to speak without first being asked, spoke up, "Sorry to interrupt you, Jimmy, but I am still confused. It is enlightening to know that there are many pox diseases, each caused by its own pox virus, but what I don't understand is how a virus that produces an animal disease, cowpox in cows, when scratched into the skin of a human being, protects that person from contracting a uniquely human disease, smallpox."

"Thank you, Sarah. It is quite obvious that I have been negligent, so I will now try to fill in the gap. Let me point out that Jenner lived before the germ theory. He knew nothing about living particles, such as viruses or bacteria, causing disease. Even without this knowledge, Jenner made an excellent guess at what was taking place. He said that when he took the poison from a cowpox lesion on the udder of a cow and inoculated it into the arm of an individual, it produced a poison in that person's body that only mildly affected him, but was capable of fighting off or neutralizing the poison in his body caused by the disease, smallpox. It is a fairly primitive answer Jenner gave, but not a bad one, when you realize that he had no other historical medical model upon which to base his conclusion. So let's see how well he did, using his imagination as his empirical model.

"Sarah, we now know that vaccination works, due to the fact that, at the molecular level, the cowpox and smallpox DNA have features that are alike. In other words, the two viruses are closely related, but not totally identical. As I said earlier, they are different species of virus belonging to the same group. We speculate that they originated from a common ancestor, hundreds of thousands of years ago.

"Once the cowpox virus is injected into the skin of a person, it reproduces itself and, at the same time, causes the immune system to produce antibodies and white blood cells which attach to the protein envelope covering the cowpox viruses, limiting their growth and eventually eliminating them. Cowpox is not a bad disease and the immune system is capable of keeping it confined to the skin at the sight of inoculation, preventing it from spreading throughout the body.

"The same antibodies and white blood cells that destroyed the cowpox viruses are also able to attack and destroy the variola or smallpox viruses, because of the common DNA sights on the protein covers of the two viruses. Simply put, the antibodies and white blood cells that protect against a cowpox infection will also protect a person from contracting smallpox.

"Sarah, I hope that explanation wasn't too long and wordy for you?" Jimmy said.

Sara replied, "No, I think that I now understand. Perhaps, by tomorrow I will have forgot, but I assure you, for now I am satisfied."

Jimmy glanced over at the Prof who gave him a stern look that amounted to "Let's get on with what you have to say about Jenner and stop all these annoying digressions."

Without further delay Jimmy continued, "After Jenner received the letter from Henry Cline...."

◆ ◆ ◆

After Jenner received the letter from Dr. Henry Cline of Lincoln's Inn Fields, confirming that vaccination made it impossible to give his patient the smallpox, there then was a series of reports from England and Europe confirming and commending Jenner's work. This was a turning point in Jenner's life, and from this time on, he would be deeply involved in defending and promoting the merits of vaccination. Despite its overwhelming success, vaccination would always have its share of defamers and defrauders.

Suddenly, there was a flood of favorable reports legitimizing Jenner's work; and just as suddenly, Dr. Ingenhousz's vituperative letters ceased. The burgeoning number of reports substantiating the correctness of his work assuaged Jenner's apprehension caused by the animosity he been subjected to, up to now.

It is of interest that one of the early verifications of vaccination occurred by chance. At the time Jenner went to London to have the *Inquiry* published, he brought some cowpox lymph with him and gave it to a colleague who was uncertain about how to use it. The doctor had a patient with a chronic hip disease which refused to heal. Wondering about the usefulness of the medicine Jenner gave him, he injected the cowpox lymph into the skin of the patient, in hopes of curing the disease. Of course, the man's chronic hip disease never healed. However, the doctor finally realized that his patient had been given cowpox disease which had successfully vaccinated him. The doctor then variolated his patient, who failed to react, proving that he was immune to smallpox, just as Jenner had predicted.

The most methodical and detailed verification of Jenner's work came in November of 1798, after Jenner left London and returned to Berkeley. The confirmation occurred at a time in Jenner's life when he was depressed and began to doubt the value of his work. Dr. George Pearson, a London doctor and teacher at St. George's Hospital, spoke with doctors throughout England who admitted to him that vaccination was responsible for preventing their patients from getting smallpox. Pearson published his findings in a report entitled, *An Inquiry Concerning the History of the Cowpox Principally with a View to Supercede and Extinguish the Smallpox*. It was this publication that did so much to confirm Jenner's discovery that vaccination worked and was a safe way of preventing smallpox.

Dr. Pearson's publication was responsible for the acceptance of vaccination, by many doctors, as the safest and best way of preventing smallpox. Unfortunately, not all the English doctors abandoned the use of variolation, and it would take another forty years before variolation was banned in England.

Dr. Pearson, an early advocate of vaccination and a friend to Jenner, soon became Jenner's adversary. It was not long after his publication, confirming Jenner's claims for vaccination, that he proclaimed that he was the true discoverer of vaccination. And it was the same Dr. Pearson who would later try to prevent Parliament from giving Jenner a financial reward for the discovery of vaccination.

But in spite of Dr. Pearson's craven acts, Jenner, the modest and enigmatic country doctor, now in his early fifties, from this time onward, would be the person known worldwide for introducing the practice of vaccination.

By the start of the year 1800, Jenner, by necessity, was forced to spend additional time in London, a city that he loathed. Jenner frequently remarked to his friends, "When I am in London, I believe in the devil; when in am in the country, I believe only in God."

In eighteenth century England, being successful depended upon acceptance by the Royal Family, and this was also true for Jenner and vaccination. The Duke of Clarence, the third oldest son of the King, was an ardent disciple of Jenner and petitioned him to attend a meeting in London, to settle a controversy at the London Vaccination Board, which had been caused by the notorious Dr. Pearson. To the Duke's delight, Jenner successfully resolved the disagreement.

The Duke, a ruling member of the Royal Navy, was so impressed with Jenner and his discovery of vaccination that he wished to have those members of the Royal Navy, who had never had smallpox, vaccinated. The Duke ordered that any cowpox lymph to be used for vaccination must meet with Jenner's approval. The infamous Dr. Pearson had been attempting to force the Royal Navy to use contaminated cowpox lymph supplied by the London Vaccination Board, which was controlled by Pearson. Even though the Duke was a man of limited intellectual abilities, he doubted Pearson's integrity, and used Jenner to defeat him.

The Duke was a powerful influence on the political and social framework of the country, albeit, he was considered a man of questionable morals. Much of the initial acceptance of vaccination by the general public, throughout the British Isles, was due to the sponsorship of the procedure by the titled nobility, such as the Duke and other members of the Royal Family—and most importantly, the King. Of almost equal significance, however, was the fact that vaccination, early on, was approved and used by both the Army and the Royal Navy.

The well justified fear of the disease, smallpox, by all populations, accounted for the universal acceptance of vaccination, once it was shown to be an effective preventative. Up until that time in medical history, no preventative medical procedure was so rapidly and extensively embraced by both the doctors and the public.

During the spring of 1799, Jenner met with Lord Egremont and the Duke of York, mainly to discuss Dr. Pearson's improper schemes related to the Vaccination Board, a continually nagging subject and a source of annoyance for Jenner.

In March, Jenner received a warrant to meet with the King, and he used the occasion to present him with the second edition of the *Inquiry*, which Jenner had dedicated to him. The book was lavishly bound and had introductory statements showing deference to the King.

Clothed in an eighteenth century velvet suit, including knickers, silk stockings covering strong, ample legs, and a sword at his waist indicative of rank and position, Jenner was escorted to St. James' Palace by his friend and patron, Lord Berkeley of Berkeley Castle.

The ceremony with the elderly King, at first, was formal and reserved. Protocol demanded that the King speak first, but once the proper etiquette was observed, Jenner was permitted to speak freely. He then proceeded to tell the King how he discovered vaccination. Less enthralled with medical discoveries than with his own preferred subject, music, the King invited Jenner's comments on the latter. Jenner assured the King of his love of music and highlighted his ability to play a variety of musical instruments. They engaged in a detailed and enjoyable discussion about concert music, the King's favorite. To further impress the King, Jenner quoted from the Ancients that, "Without music, life would be a mistake." Shortly thereafter, the interview ended. Jenner's high-spirited personality delighted the King.

Lord Berkeley and Jenner were about to retire from the Royal Chamber, but only after the King first withdrew to return to his private quarters.

Eighteenth century England was the time of the Enlightenment, and the King recognized Jenner as a leader in the movement. Later, the King told Queen Charlotte about the exciting and progressive Dr. Jenner whom he had interviewed. Some time later, Queen Charlotte summoned Jenner for an interview and requested a copy of his newest book. Jenner and vaccination were now strongly approved among the Royal Family, and consequently, they were accepted by most of the English nobility and the general public.

And then there was the handsome and dashing General Charles O'Hara and the lovely Mary Berry. Both made a contribution to the acceptance of vaccination as the most appropriate way of preventing smallpox. He was one of the first generals to popularize vaccination in the English military; she introduced vaccination into Ireland.

Before he knew anything about vaccination, O'Hara was romantically involved with Mary Berry, at the time, one of England's most beautiful women. Mary was young, vivacious and just the sort of woman that the brave and spirited General O'Hara would have found attractive. And because they both performed an essential part in the history of vaccination, it is necessary to tell their stories.

Mary was first known to Jenner about 1795, much before he published the *Inquiry*. He had recently bought a house and established a part-time medical practice in Cheltenham, while still maintaining his home and medical practice in Berkeley.

Mary was in her mid-twenties and had grown up in a family of modest resources, but due to her physical beauty and natural endowments, she and her sister soon were invited into the wealthy society that frequented Cheltenham. Being beautiful wasn't Mary's only attribute; she was also highly intelligent and a gifted authoress. Lord Orford and his family esteemed it an honor to have Mary visit with them in their summer home in Cheltenham, and she soon became their permanent house guest. As you can imagine, Mary had many admirers, the most famous and well-known was General Charles O'Hara. Before long, he came to occupy all her time and soon declared his love for her, affirming some sort of vague intention of marrying her. All the time, he knew full well that he soon would be off to France, in the service of his country.

Unbeknownst to Mary, the General was a bit of a rogue, with a history of unsavory affairs with other women. Before leaving for France, he made some imprecise commitment to Mary, in hopes that she would agree to a sexual liaison, but Mary was wary, telling him it would have to wait until they were married.

In France, during the siege of Toulon, the general was captured and sent to Paris during the Reign of Terror. He was later released, during an exchange of prisoners, and returned to Cheltenham.

Back in Cheltenham, the General was the toast of the city, a real hero who entertained at numerous dinner parties that were arranged for him. Everyone was intrigued by the fact that he had been a captive and lived to tell about it. In Cheltenham, O'Hara joined Jenner's cadre of aristocratic and intellectual friends. The General captivated his select audience with exciting tales of his capture by the French. Especially stimulating was his forced stay in Lyons where he was compelled to remain by Dr. Guillotin's ungainly and barbaric invention, La Guillotine. The General related, in intimate detail, how he was forced to watch the sharp edge of the blade decapitate nearly forty persons, some of them young girls under the age of fifteen, never knowing if he would be the next victim of "Madam Guillotine." His companions were enthralled by his tales of horror. With great emotion and empathy, the General told his story. He went into minute detail in the telling of the executions and serial sadistic behavior that he was subjected to, while a prisoner. His audiences, especially the ladies, were appalled by his tales; nevertheless, they beseeched him to press on with his stories.

Jenner, on one of these social occasions, was among the few guests. He tried to accept the General's tale objectively without becoming too emotionally involved. Another of the guests that evening was Mary Berry who sat and gazed at the General with admiration and approbation, as he talked.

The purpose for the General's visit to Cheltenham, upon being freed from his French prison was, of course, to see Mary. Since O'Hara made his pretense of marriage before leaving for France, Mary expected that she and the General would soon be wed. Any commitment he made to Mary, before leaving for France, was in secret and never made public. While O'Hara had returned with amorous plans for a relationship before marriage, Mary still would have none of it, until after the wedding ceremony.

Never to be out-done, the indomitable and morally unrestrained General begged Mary to spend twenty-four hours with him in London, before he departed for his new posting. Prudently, Mary denied him his one last request. The debonair and dapper General then left Mary with her virginity and innocence still intact, while he shipped out of her life forever on a schooner for Gibraltar. Eventually, the not so gentlemanly General, soon lost all interest in Mary. When he arrived in Gibraltar, he quickly consoled himself over the loss of Mary by acquiring two mistresses with whom he produced numerous children. As it turned out, the General seemed to have been short on virtues and long on vices.

While the General may have quickly forgotten about Mary Berry, he always remembered Dr. Jenner. The high-spirited General was appointed Governor of Gibraltar, and he immediately advocated the use of Jenner's discovery in the colony, by having the troops vaccinated. The English government supported his position on vaccination and quickly proposed the use of vaccination in Malta. While the General turned out to be less than an honest lover, he was quick to recognize the value of vaccination, in the military, and its desirability in confined areas such as Gibraltar and Malta. It wasn't long afterwards that the General suddenly died on Gibraltar, his death having gone almost unnoticed in the English army, and his contributions passed unrewarded by history.

Mary Berry remained somewhat the wiser, and a part of Cheltenham society, until the day she died. She held Jenner in the highest esteem, and continued to champion vaccination all her life. Not to be discomfited by General O'Hara, Mary was responsible for the introduction and acceptance of vaccination in Ireland. And while General O'Hara died at a relatively young age, Mary lived a long and happy life and died still a maiden.

King George III and his entourage visited Cheltenham, after his first attack of insanity. It was but a short visit, and soon after he left, he had a more serious second attack, about which there were differences of opinion concerning its cause. Some blamed the second attack on his visit to the spa, while others suggested that, if he had remained at Cheltenham, the second attack would not have occurred. But the very fact that the King visited the spa for his health, and his entourage indulged themselves in the spa and drank the healing waters was, to a large extent, the reason for the town becoming a center of the summer social season. It became equal in importance to the historic Roman spa at Bath. Not only did Royalty build their summer homes there, but the aristocracy and the wealthy followed suit.

Dr. Jenner had the highest regard for the Cheltenham waters, but he lamented that the waters could be taken unwisely and excessively, the results of which were especially noticeable in the bloated facial features of some of the young ladies.

As Jenner pointed out to a friend, "So far this season, about three thousand persons have quenched their thirst or bathed in the waters of the spa, and not one of them who came for its benefits has died." For Jenner, Cheltenham was a place for socializing and intellectual excitement, since it was frequented by painters, poets and musicians. The highlight of many of the evening gatherings was the presence of the delightful and intelligent Berry sisters. But of Jenner's many new friends, one of his favorites was the internationally famous Irish tenor, Michael Kelly.

Jenner's life was dedicated to the welfare of all mankind, and the publication of the *Inquiry* was the culmination of this dedication. From foreign countries, there was an endless request for cowpox lymph and instructions how to use it. In most countries, public vaccinations were of the utmost priority. Initially, Jenner attempted to fulfill all these demands. He mailed cowpox lymph samples, at his own expense, and wrote letters of instructions to anyone requesting his aid. Jenner was meticulous in the collection of the lymph so that spurious or contaminated samples would not be sent by mistake. All this was time consuming and expensive, so much so, that he no longer had time to care for his patients in Berkeley or Cheltenham. All these things put a strain on his finances which he could ill afford.

Jenner could have become a rich man, had he wished. He could have kept the knowledge of vaccination a secret and offered to vaccinate wealthy patients for exorbitant fees. Furthermore, he could have charged large fees, to anyone requesting cowpox lymph for vaccination. Being a man true to his science, and conforming to what he considered the moral principles of good medicine, he made known his discovery and supplied his cowpox lymph and instructions how to use it free to everyone who requested them.

20

SO FAR IT HAD BEEN A LONG NIGHT, but all agreed a productive one. The Prof, the oldest of the group, though, as usual, was still ebullient and overflowing with enthusiasm for his subject. "*By God!*" he thought to himself, "*I started this discussion and I'll see to it that we'll finish it before this night is over.*" How his tired gathering would have reacted to such a remark is not known, but, on the surface, it appeared they were physically prepared to carry on—for a while, at least.

"Valerie!" he interjected, almost as a stimulant, "it is known that in your country, vaccination was quickly accepted as the treatment of choice for preventing smallpox. Jenner's publication, the *Inquiry*, arrived there, nearly a year after it was first published in England. While in England, there were many doctors who denied both Jenner and vaccination, yet, in the United States, he was acknowledged as a hero and worshipped for what he had accomplished. How can you explain the difference?"

"Prof, we know that the Indian tribes throughout the New World were ravaged by smallpox, but at the same time, the settlers were also perishing in large numbers from the same demon, smallpox, that many classified as 'the most terrible of all the ministers of death.' And this was only one of the many foul epithets attributed to smallpox; still, it does reflect the fear and trepidation the new settlers had for the disease.

"For years, the English people heard the stories of wealth, and, in some cases, religious freedom, that existed in this 'New World.' By the seventeenth century there were many people ready to go and tame the reputed wilderness. They failed to realized, however, that once they arrived at this utopia, medically, things would be worse than where they came from.

"For example, in 1607, the first permanent English settlement was established in Jamestown, Virginia, and a variety of diseases, including smallpox, caused many more deaths to the settlers than all the Indian raids combined. It is difficult to realize how bad their conditions were, and what a large proportion of the population was susceptible to disease. For example, in 1610, of the 398 people living in the colony, 338 died of smallpox and other diseases—an 85% death rate in one year.

"The Puritans in New England suffered a similar fate. At first, they gloated that God must be on their side, since disease had destroyed so many of the Indians, thus making room for them to expand. At any rate, their rejoicing didn't last long, for in the early months of 1621, the same diseases that overwhelmed the Jamestown colonists attacked the Puritans, with smallpox, 'the destroyer of mankind,' leading the group. It wasn't long before half the population of Massachusetts had died.

"And so it was, through the entire 17th century. As the colonists expanded along the east coast of the continent, death due to disease was the monster that they had to tame, and not the guiltless Indians. And by the beginning of the eighteenth century, as one English historian wrote, 'the smallpox was ever present, filling the church yards with corpses, tormenting with the constant fear all whom it had not yet stricken...turning the babe into a changeling at which the mother shuddered.'

"In some parts of the country, smallpox visited only periodically, but places like New York, New Jersey and Pennsylvania were rarely free of the disease. Yet, certain of the southern colonies seemed to be better off, since they were only infrequently visited by smallpox. It was thought their isolation and scattered populations prevented the spread of the disease.

"Boston, on the other hand, was tormented by smallpox, having had a series of prolonged epidemics of the disease starting at the beginning of the eighteenth century. And smallpox was endemic throughout the revolutionary War. It was in Boston that the British attempted to use smallpox as a form of biological warfare against the colonial army of George Washington.

"During the smallpox epidemic, of 1736, in Philadelphia, the sagacious Benjamin Franklin lost his four-year-old son to smallpox. The boy's grave, which I visited, is still to be found in downtown Philadelphia.

"Anyway, Prof, smallpox ravaged the English colonies throughout the seventeenth and eighteenth centuries, right up until the time Jenner published the results of his remarkable discovery. Is it any wonder then that vaccination was greeted with such enthusiasm, when the people in the United States heard about it? Vaccination proved to be such a simple and effective tool for preventing the disease. It is understandable why Jenner was greeted as a hero in the United States."

"Fine, Valerie. I'm sure that we can all visualize what smallpox had bestowed on these bewildered peoples; now, perhaps, you can quickly tells us what happened to them after 1798, when they learned of Jenner and his new treatment, vaccination."

"While the practice of vaccination...."

◆ ◆ ◆

While the practice of vaccination was rapidly spreading throughout Europe and Asia, the Americas were not far behind them. The first place in North America to receive the vaccine was Newfoundland. By vaccinating small children in sequence, on the six weeks it took the ship to cross the ocean from England, the vaccine, supplied by Jenner, arrived safely.

It was nearly a year after the *Inquiry* was published before Dr. John Coakley Lettsom, of the United States, received his copy. He immediately recognized its importance and forwarded the *Inquiry* on to Dr. Benjamin Waterhouse, Professor of the Theory and Practice of Physic at the Harvard Medical School, Cambridge, Massachusetts.

In 1783, Dr. Waterhouse, together with two other professors, had established the Harvard Medical School. After reading the *Inquiry,* as well as the copies of Pearson's publication on Vaccination, and Woodville's Experiments, that were included with it, Waterhouse was impressed and grasped the significance of what Jenner had accomplished when he discovered vaccination.

Waterhouse, along with Thomas Jefferson (1743–1826), the third president of the United States—whose life spans overlapped that of Jenner's—were the two men who did the most to advance the practice of vaccination in the United States.

Waterhouse was so excited by what he had read that he quickly wrote an article for a Boston newspaper describing Jenner's discovery. Unfortunately, the article received little attention. Since there was no cowpox in the dairy herds in America, the public failed to grasp the significance of Waterhouse's article. For the public, variolation was the only way of preventing smallpox.

Waterhouse next decided to present Jenner's discovery at a meeting of the American Academy of Arts and Sciences, an organization better prepared to understand the importance of what Jenner had accomplished. The academy membership included John Adams (1735–1826), the president of the Academy, who, at the same time, was President of the United States. Waterhouse's report on vaccination was accepted with great enthusiasm. President Adams, the second president of the United States, understood the significance of the report and quickly became one of vaccination's greatest enthusiasts.

Not only did Waterhouse write and lecture about vaccination, he requested vaccine from Jenner with which to vaccinate his family. After several unsuccessful attempts at sending vaccine on the six weeks' journey across the ocean, Waterhouse finally received cowpox-impregnated thread in suitable condition for performing vaccinations. Although he had seven children, he elected, for whatever reason, to first experiment on one child, his five-year-old son. He recorded the details: "The first of my children that I inoculated (vaccinated) was a boy of five years old, named Daniel Oliver Waterhouse. I made a slight incision in the usual place for inoculation (vaccination) in the arm, inserted a small portion of the infected thread, and covered it with a sticking plaster."

Today what Waterhouse did seems routine and ordinary, but for the doctor, it was adventuring into new and unexplored areas of medical knowledge. Most assuredly, he experienced the worry and apprehension that goes along with taking such a big step.

The boy's medical course closely followed that described in the *Inquiry*, and by the eighth day, he showed the typical signs of a vaccination reaction. Waterhouse's apprehension was relieved when he observed, "the sore on the boy's arm looked just like the second drawing in Jenner's book."

Satisfied vaccination was as safe as Jenner reported. Waterhouse then proceeded to vaccinate his remaining six children, using cowpox lymph taken from the cowpox pustule on Daniel's arm. In addition to his own children, Waterhouse vaccinated the children of his household staff. All the children went through the experience of vaccination with little or no interference in their daily routines. These were the first vaccinations done in the United States.

To verify that cowpox vaccine, which in the United States was referred to as kine-pock, truly prevented smallpox, Waterhouse invited the assistance of a Dr. William Aspinwall, a doctor at the smallpox hospital in Boston, to variolate a 12 years-old boy, whom he previously had vaccinated. As Waterhouse describes what happened: "The Dr. chose to try the experiment on the boy of 12 years of age…whom he inoculated in my presence by two punctures, and with matter taken that moment from a patient who had it (smallpox) pretty full upon in. He at the same time inserted an infected thread, and then put him (the boy) into the hospital, where was one patient with it (smallpox) the natural way. On the 4th day, the Dr. pronounced the arm to be infected. It became every hour sorer but in a day or two it dried off, and grew well; so that the boy was dismissed from the hospital and returned home the 12th day after the experiment."

The experiment was a success and it proved that the boy was immune to smallpox after being vaccinated, just as Jenner had recorded in the *Inquiry*.

Waterhouse was such an ardent enthusiast of vaccination that, by 1800, he was referred to as the "Jenner of America." In the same year, he wrote, "I was struck with the unspeakable advantages that might accrue to this country, and indeed to the human race at large, from the discovery of a mild distemper (vaccination) that would ever after secure the constitution from that terrible scourge, the smallpox."

The first publication in the United States on vaccination was written by Waterhouse titled, *A Prospect of Exterminating the Small-Pox*.

Some of the doctors in the Boston area resented Waterhouse's vigorous support of vaccination and, in 1802, requested the City Board of Health to do an evaluation study on both vaccination and variolation. To the dismay of the dissident doctors, vaccination was shown to be the superior of the two and its use was recommended by the Board. Later, these same doctors denigrated Waterhouse for not sharing his vaccine supply with them and for demanding a share of their profits when he did. It was at this time that Waterhouse had the only supply of live vaccine, which he planned to control, until, in his own mind, he was convinced that vaccination was all that Jenner claimed it to be. In the meantime, because vaccination had become the craze, his major fear was taking place. Quacks and charlatans, realizing that there was money to be made, were selling spurious cowpox lymph for the real thing. Waterhouse stated the problem clearly when he wrote: "During this period, viz., the autumn of 1800, a singular traffic was carried on in the article of kine-pock matter (cowpox), by persons not in the least connected with the medical profession; such as stage-drivers, pedlars (peddlers) and in one instance the sexton of a church. I have known the shirt sleeve of a patient stiff with the purulent discharge from a foul ulcer made so by unskillful management, and full three weeks after vaccination, and in which there could have been none of the specific virus; I have known this cut up into small strips, and sold about the country as genuine kine-pock (cowpox) matter, coming directly from me. Several hundred people were inoculated (vaccinated) with this caustic morbid poison, which produced great inflammation, sickness fever, and in severe cases, eruptions."

Waterhouse's major worry was that he couldn't persuade those who were swindled that they were not really vaccinated and were still able to contract smallpox. The reason such egregious practices were able to occur was that vaccination was extremely popular. The popularity occurred after he published his glowing reports on the procedure.

Still, Waterhouse himself wasn't totally satisfied, and he wanted additional information that his conclusions about vaccination were valid. He devised additional experiments in order to verify that vaccination really prevented smallpox. Unfortunately, his first attempt ended as a disaster. Waterhouse, with the aid of another doctor, vaccinated a group of children with lymph taken from the arm of a sailor, who assured Waterhouse's assistant that what he had were cowpox lesions. The lesions, it turned out, were those of smallpox, and a number of the children inoculated with this material died. In addition, a smallpox epidemic occurred in the community. This was just the kind of accident that Waterhouse had hoped to prevent, but, in the early days of vaccination in the United States, such mishaps were common and people were soon beginning to lose faith in the procedure.

Still, Waterhouse had previously had success with his experiments. He had vaccinated 12 children and then decided to variolate them in order to prove that they were immune to smallpox. He noted that: "The small-pox matter excited no general indisposition whatever, through the whole progress of the experiments, though the children took no medicines but were indulged in their usual modes of living and exercise, and were all lodged promiscuously in one room."

Nevertheless, Waterhouse wanted even more proof of the efficacy of vaccination. So with the same smallpox lymph that he used on the 12 boys to prove that they were immune to smallpox, he inoculated or variolated an additional two boys, who previously had neither cowpox nor smallpox. Both boys showed a positive reaction to the smallpox inoculation; namely, they developed classical smallpox lesions, thus proving that the smallpox lymph he used was truly infectious, containing active smallpox particles. Finally, he was able to show, to his own satisfaction, and that of all his medical colleagues, that vaccination truly protected against that frightful scourge smallpox, just as Jenner had predicted it would.

Waterhouse's main desire was to assure himself and others that vaccination was, first of all, safe and also capable of preventing smallpox. However, there were those at Harvard who attempted to blacken his good name and ruin his reputation because he charged a fee to other doctors for supplying them with the cowpox vaccine supplied to him by Jenner.

It was unfortunate that in-house political intrigue and jealousy at Harvard overshadowed the attributes of an honest and decent doctor. Waterhouse, unfortunately, was dismissed from the Harvard Medical School and forced to relinquish his faculty position as professor. However, integrity and honesty finally carried the day for Waterhouse, because he continued to champion the cause of vaccination, and in doing so, over the years, he was directly and indirectly responsible for saving millions the lives in the United States. Luckily, Waterhouse was able to continue his distinguished medical career after leaving Harvard Medical School, and at the end of his life, he was known as one of the founding fathers of American medicine.

It was also to Waterhouse's credit the he was the one who introduced Thomas Jefferson to the new vaccination technique discovered by Jenner. Jefferson became one of vaccination's most ardent proponents. He later wrote to Waterhouse, in his inimitable writing style, that "Every friend of humanity must look with pleasure on this discovery, by which one more evil is withdrawn from the condition of man." It is remarkable how all three men, Jenner, Waterhouse and Jefferson, recognized the advantages of vaccination, not only for the individual, but for all mankind as well; and in their writings acknowledged, in a furtive manner, that, some day, smallpox could be eliminated from all mankind.

After receiving the vaccine from Waterhouse, Jefferson vaccinated his family members, plantation slaves, and two hundred of his Virginia neighbors, as well as providing vaccine for several of the local Indian tribes. In 1804, Jefferson also secured cowpox vaccine for the Lewis and Clark expedition, with which he hoped they would vaccinate the west coast Indian tribes, when they arrived there.

Jefferson was a great admirer of Jenner, and held him in the highest esteem for his discovery of vaccination. It was Jefferson, more than anyone else in the United States, who understood that such a malignant disease as smallpox could destroy the fabric of the country and delay it from achieving its stately destiny. In a letter to Jenner in 1806, Jefferson, in his unique prose, expressed his gratitude: "Future generations will know by history only that the loathsome smallpox existed and by you has been extirpated." When Jenner died in 1823, it was Jefferson who acknowledged that: "he (Jenner) was the most honored man of his age."

Another early vaccinator was a controversial doctor named James Smith of Baltimore. Smith became involved in public health matters in Baltimore, in 1797, when he defied the Baltimore Board of Health by announcing to the local newspaper that a serious yellow fever epidemic was present in the city. His announcement was made much to the annoyance of the Board of Health and the City Fathers, who were trying to cover-up the epidemic, since it would be bad for business.

Dr. Smith later was appointed doctor to the county almshouse and, in 1801, performed the first vaccination in the city of Baltimore on a seven-year-old girl, and later vaccinated many young children that were wards of the city. He offered to share his vaccine with other physicians in the city, but none of them accepted his offer. However, after publishing the results of his vaccinations, the Medical and Chirurgical Faculty of Maryland gave approval of and support for his work.

Later, the city gave its consent for Dr. Smith to establish a vaccination clinic in his home, in order to make vaccine available to everyone and to guarantee that the vaccine was pure and administered properly. This was the first vaccination clinic in the United States, and it was later copied in other parts of the country, as a model. Smith's zeal was so great for Jenner's remarkable discovery that he named his child, Edward Jenner Smith, in honor of the great English doctor.

In 1813, Congress sanctioned President James Madison (1751–1836) to appoint Dr. Smith as the agent to maintain the purity of the vaccine being furnished to anyone requesting it in the United States. The program was such a great success that Smith was later permitted to supply the vaccine to anyone requesting it, in the western hemisphere. He was eventually credited with supplying vaccine to the American military during the War of 1812. Afterwards he was commended for preventing serious smallpox epidemics occurring during that campaign.

At the same time that Jenner was sending vaccine to the United States, the Vaccination Institute at Bath, England was also shipping vaccine to the New England area, particularly the State of Massachusetts. Cowpox did not occur naturally in the cattle herds of North or South America so it had to be shipped in from England or some European countries. When the vaccine arrived from Bath, a number of small children were immediately vaccinated to determine if the vaccine was still useable after such a long journey. If the vaccine were still good, then the children would be immune to smallpox. The test to determine if the vaccine worked was to variolate, that is to inoculate the skin on the arm of a few of the children with smallpox virus, and if they failed to get sick or develop smallpox pustules, they then were immune to smallpox. When it was finally demonstrated that all these children were protected against the dreaded smallpox, there was the satisfaction of achievement and accomplishment. But, unfortunately, the rejoicing didn't last long. Soon there were doubts being expressed about the merits of vaccination, since, later on, individuals who had been vaccinated developed smallpox.

It was a frightening failure and a significant reversal for the practice of vaccination. Fortunately, there were two important individuals who correctly guessed what had happened to cause such a major mishap. Interestingly enough, they were two of the early American presidents, John Adams and Thomas Jefferson. They surmised correctly that improper handling by the vaccinators enabled the cowpox vaccine, shipped in good condition from Bath, to become contaminated by the smallpox virus, sometime after it had arrived in Massachusetts. Regrettably this was a common, unfortunate accident, during the early days of vaccination in the United States, as well as in England and Europe. Doctors and other vaccinators, inexperienced in the care and use of the vaccine, caused the smallpox virus to contaminate their stock of cowpox vaccine. It was something that both Jenner and Waterhouse predicted would happen, if the individuals doing the vaccinating were not properly trained or experienced. Jenner, when he shipped his vaccine abroad, sent with it a set of detailed written instructions on the care and use of the material.

The Massachusetts misadventure was solved by destroying their vaccine and requesting that the Vaccination Institute at Bath supply them with a new supply of cowpox vaccine.

It is no small matter that three of the early presidents of the United States, John Adams, Thomas Jefferson and James Madison were knowledgeable about and actively engaged in the promotion of vaccination as the proper way to control smallpox. The also realized that for the country to grow and reach it greatest potential there had to be universal vaccinations. The presidents all acknowledged Jenner for his important contribution to mankind.

Transporting the vaccine long distances, especially across oceans, was a problem, especially when it was going to a hot and humid climate. Vaccines, in sealed containers, being shipped to South America and parts of North America, were frequently degraded by the time they reached their destinations. The Americas depended on England and Spain for their supplies of cowpox vaccine, since cowpox did not occur naturally on either of the continents.

Jenner was able to show that the vaccine could be successfully kept alive in a quill, or on a thread saturated with lymph from a cowpox lesion, and sealed in a glass container. The problem was that both methods of transportation had serious limitations. The vaccine would remain viable (active) for only a limited time and high temperatures appreciably affected its survivability.

As part of Jenner's initial experiments, he demonstrated that the vaccine could be kept active by doing serial vaccinations, which involved removing lymph from the vaccination sight of one individual and using this same lymph to vaccinate another individual. Theoretically, if the procedure was carried out with care, the lymph (vaccine) could be transferred indefinitely from on individual to another.

Serial vaccination was the method elected by the Spanish to transport the vaccine to their colonies in Mexico, Central and South America and the Caribbean Islands. Serial vaccinations were used quite successfully on board Spanish vessels. Young children were selected that had never been vaccinated or exposed to smallpox. At the beginning of each voyage two children were vaccinated and after crusted lesions formed at the vaccination site, lymph was removed and used to vaccinate two additional children. Two children were always vaccinated at the same time, in case one of the vaccines failed there would still be lymph available to continue on with the serial vaccinations.

In 1802, the Spanish ruler, King Carlos IV, was troubled about the smallpox epidemics occurring in his vast overseas colonies. Carlos knew of Jenner and he had even read the *Inquiry*. Subsequently, he had his three children vaccinated. Later, he acknowledged that vaccination was responsible for saving his daughter's life, after she was exposed to the disease.

For the welfare of his subjects, Carlos was determined to establish vaccination in his part of the New World. His problem was how to keep the vaccine alive during the long ocean voyages to his colonies. These colonies stretched for thousands of miles across a vast ocean. The standard methods of transporting the vaccine were in quills or saturating threads with cowpox lymph. These methods frequently failed, under the hash conditions of distance and high temperatures that were encountered to reach his colonies.

Carlos' medical advisor, Jose Felipe de Flores, proposed they use serial vaccination of young children, who previously had neither smallpox nor cowpox, as the best way to transport the vaccine.

Flores determined that on the tenth day after vaccination, sufficient lymph could be removed from the initial vaccination sight with which to vaccinate two additional children. With an adequate number of children on board the vessel, he could continue serial vaccinations until the ship reached its destination. Prior to this, the use of serial vaccinations over such a long distances was untested. Flores, therefore, prudently decided to also transport the vaccine by other methods as a precaution. A few cows were infected with cowpox disease and were brought aboard the ship to make the long trip. Flores was a cautious man and also brought along vaccine samples, sealed in glass containers, just in case all else failed. Trusting in God and his own reasoning, and with some good luck in the mix, Flores hoped that one of the three methods for transporting the vaccine would prevail and it would arrive in the New World in good condition.

The ship sailed from Corunna, Spain with 26 young children to be used in the serial vaccination experiment. After a very long voyage and numerous serial vaccinations, the expedition arrived safely in Puerto Rico with the vaccine intact. In Puerto Rico, the vaccine and the children were divided and put on board two separate ships. One ship proceeded to Buenos Aires and the other ship to Havana and Mexico, with their precious cargoes of vaccine and children.

Dr. Jose Felipe de Flores was both a lucky and a clever man who later got the Pope to agree to approve the coupling of vaccination with the ceremony of baptism, thus removing any religious opposition to the practice of vaccination.

In Spanish America, it was later claimed, smallpox had been eliminated as the result of the vaccination programs initiated by the Spanish.

21

"IT IS ABSOLUTELY AMAZING—PERHAPS, I should say almost unbelievable—the speed with which the practice of vaccination spread around the world, when the fastest forms of transportation, at that time, were the horse and sailing ship," the Prof offered, while at the same time, shaking his head from side-to-side, in disbelief.

"I believe the swiftness with which vaccination was accepted around the world was an indication of the need for a better way of protecting people against smallpox than variolation, which was then being used in many countries," Murray said. "Turkey is a good example of what I am talking about. As you remember, it was in Turkey that Lady Montagu first learned about variolation, or, as it was referred to there, smallpox inoculation or 'buying the pock.' Buying the pock existed since ancient times in Turkey. It was a custom going back hundreds of years and was well accepted in the country. Nevertheless, when Dr. de Carro sent cowpox vaccine to the British embassy in Constantinople, and vaccination was introduced among the English population stationed there, it wasn't long before it was also accepted by the Turkish population, and the ancient practice of buying the pock was discontinued."

"I'm sure that you are correct, Murray," the Prof said as a way of encouraging him to continue.

Murray carefully considered what he wanted to say, for the use of proper English, whether written or spoken, was of the utmost importance to Murray. This evening would be a total disaster, if his subject and verb did not agree in number.

Finally, after only seconds, but what seemed to the other guests, including his wife, as an agonizingly long time, Murray began, "Perhaps, at the time, how to successfully transport the vaccine long distances, and still keep it alive, was the most formidable problem."

Cedric saw an opening and jumped in, much to Murray's chagrin. "You must remember, it was Jenner who was first faced with this problem, and he did a damn good job of getting the ball rolling."

Murray, upset by the one-upmanship game that Cedric insisted on playing, whether at the university, or at a private gathering such as this evening, replied, "I thought that you felt Jenner was getting too much credit, and now, I hear you championing his cause!"

The Prof could not allow this type of discussion to continue so he interrupted, "Come, come, gentlemen! A little civility, please. Now, back to the topic of transporting the cowpox vaccine."

Cedric continued. "As the requests for vaccine increased from various parts of the world, new methods for transporting it were improvised. For example, when de Carro saw the need to send the vaccine to other countries, he employed a method conceived by a Dr. Ballhorn who devised a new and better method for protecting the vaccine. Two glass plates were used—one was flat and the second plate had a concave surface in the center, forming a well to hold the vaccine. The vaccine was placed in the concave well and was covered with the flat plate. At first, the edges were merely sealed by daubing them with oil; later, they were permanently sealed by covering the edges with layer-on-layer of wax.

"For long sea voyages, as we have just learned, the Spanish used serial vaccinations of young children to keep the vaccine alive, a procedure that was quite successful.

"The methods of storing and transporting the vaccine went unchanged until the mid-nineteenth century when a new method of preserving the vaccine was introduced in Naples, Italy, in 1834. A Dr. Negri showed that by infecting healthy cows with cowpox, he could maintain an adequate supply of the vaccine, thus making serial vaccinations in humans unnecessary.

"By 1866, the French improved on Negri's method, by using heifers instead of cows. For a long time, the vaccine was produced by shaving the belly and inner thighs of a calf and inoculating the skin of these areas with the cowpox virus. Eight days later, crusts formed and were collected. The vaccine material was accumulated and was then freeze-dried and stored until needed. Theoretically, the freeze-dried material would remain in good condition indefinitely. In order to reconstitute the freeze-dried material, a wetting agent was added to the vial, just prior to using it.

"Vaccination, fortunately, has had it lighter moments too. 'Punch,' the British humor magazine, in 1881 published the following:

> 'To vaccinate or not, that is the question!
> Whether 'tis better for a man to suffer
> The painful pangs and lasting scars of smallpox,
> Or to bare arms before the surgeon's lancet,
> And by being vaccinated, end them. Yes!
> To see the tiny point, and say we end
> The chance of many a thousand awful scars
> That flesh is heir to—'tis a consummation
> Devoutly to be wished. Ah! Soft, you, now,
> The vaccinator! Sir, upon thy rounds
> Be my poor arm remembered.'

Cedric continued, "It wasn't long after...."

◆ ◆ ◆

It wasn't long after the *Inquiry* was published and translated into many languages, before the use of vaccination began to spread around the world. Soon afterwards, a multitude of reports, from many different countries, began to be received by Jenner, confirming his original contention that vaccination prevented smallpox. Along with the affirmative reports, came expressions of approval and admiration for Jenner himself. Undoubtedly, Jenner relished the commendations, but he was a modest enough man not to revel in them as a reflection of his own personal achievement; instead, he was delighted that vaccination was such an extraordinarily successful method of preventing smallpox. But most of all, he derived a great deal of satisfaction from the fact that vaccination was now saving so many lives, far more than he imagined, over thirty-years earlier, when he first began to think about cowpox and the dairymaids.

Dr. de Carro, Jenner's first European contact, wrote him from Vienna, in September of 1799. The doctor was originally from Geneva, Switzerland but, for the past six years, he had practiced medicine in Vienna. He explained that he could communicate with Jenner in English, without difficulty, since he obtained his medical degree from the University of Edinburgh in Scotland. Recently, he had the honor of reading the *Inquiry* and was excited by the results of vaccination. He then explained that he had received some cowpox vaccine, from a Dr. Pearson in London, with which he carried out several vaccinations; some were successful, while others were not.

In glowing terms, he recounted how he was confident that Jenner's vaccination procedure would be of great value to mankind. However, his immediate problem was that he had no vaccine and there was no cowpox in the cow herds of Austria. H asked Jenner to please send him a supply of vaccine through the British Legation in Vienna, and Jenner immediately did so.

Very soon, Jenner began receiving many such letters from around the world, but de Carro's letters were special. In them, he projected an enthusiasm that was astonishing, and he expressed the same great emotion for vaccination as did Jenner himself. It was this same wonderful passion that enabled de Carro to disseminate information about vaccination throughout France, Holland, Sweden, Turkey, Iraq and finally, India.

De Carro and Jenner exchanged letters for many years, always about vaccination; never once did either doctor presume to engage the other in more personal topics. For de Carro, such behavior was understandable, for he held Jenner in such high esteem that he deemed it would be a breech of etiquette to engage him in a personal manner. But such aloofness by Jenner was unusual, especially with a colleague who had done so much to advance the cause of vaccination.

Jenner was, by now, in his early fifties and the effects of aging and his new universal obligations were starting to impose a toll on him. In addition, Jenner, who loved his wife dearly, now had to watch her wither away as the result of her protracted and debilitating disease, pulmonary tuberculosis.

Surprisingly, Jenner received a package from a doctor in Hamburg, Germany which contained a copy of his *Inquiry* that had been translated into Latin. Enclosed with the publication was a letter, also in Latin, praising and complimenting Jenner and using the salutation, "The very great man, Jenner." The contents of the letter assured him that vaccination was well established in Germany. Sometime later, through diplomatic channels, Jenner received another letter from Germany, but this time it was from a Princess Louisa of Prussia requesting a supply of vaccine. Jenner promptly fulfilled her request. By this time, he was supplying vaccine, along with a personal handwritten letter of instruction on the proper use and care of his cowpox vaccine, to anyone around the world requesting his help. The Prussian doctors who were the actual recipients of the Princess' request were pleased and, in 1800, they established the Royal Vaccination Institution in Berlin.

In the meantime, de Carro continued his activities in Europe preaching the virtues of vaccination and supplying the vaccine to anyone requesting it. He supplied a friend, a Dr. Odier, in Geneva, Switzerland with the vaccine, and within a year's time, Dr. Odier completed 1500 successful vaccinations, published scientific articles on the value of vaccination, and had the Health Department distribute leaflets to the public entitled: *Advice to Fathers and Mothers*, which was given to parents, when they had their infants baptized. By combining vaccination with the practice of baptism, the procedure received religious approval and assured that the infant would eventually be vaccinated.

But the energetic and enigmatic de Carro did not stop there, for soon he was busy introducing vaccination into Hungary, Poland, Russia, Venice and Lombardy. Being able to supply cowpox vaccine to all his new contacts was getting to be a major problem for the good doctor, but in Lombardy, he became lucky, for it was there that de Carro joined forces with a determined doctor like himself, a Dr. Sacco. At a time when the need for cowpox vaccine was acute, the indomitable Dr. Sacco discovered that cowpox was present among the cow herds of Lombardy; this assured that the two doctors had an unlimited supply of the precious cowpox vaccine. With an unlimited supply of vaccine available, the Milan Vaccine Institute was established, and Dr. Sacco was appointed its director with the title of Director of Vaccination for the Cisalpine Republic. From Italy, the practice of vaccination spread along the Dalmation coast, and on into Greece.

Reports on the successes of vaccination continued to be received by Jenner. Denmark, for example, in 1810, made vaccination compulsory for all its citizens, while simultaneously banning smallpox inoculations, viz. variolation. For the following nine years, no cases of smallpox were reported in the country. From Denmark, vaccination moved to Sweden, where it was made mandatory in 1811.

Russia was infested with the terrifying villain, smallpox. For years, smallpox inoculation, variolation, was practiced, yet one in seven of those variolated died of smallpox. The Dowager Empress, humiliated by what was happening in Russia, and willing to accept Dr. de Carro's bidding, ordered that the first infant to be vaccinated be named Vaccinoff. The infant rode in a coach, in jubilation, to St. Petersburg, and received a pension for life. Had Jenner been there, he too would have received great honors and rewards. However, he was given a title, which he promptly rejected on the grounds that he lacked the necessary financial means of living up to such a position. To make amends, the Dowager Empress, in a letter, expressed her gratitude and that of the Russian people for what Jenner had accomplished for them. Enclosed with the letter was a diamond ring sent to Jenner as a personal gift from the Empress. Russia became an ardent proponent of vaccination and mandated that, within three years, the entire population be vaccinated.

But there was no head of state that showed greater admiration for Jenner than Napoleon Bonaparte of France. As the supreme ruler of the French Empire and General of the French Armies, he had good reasons for respecting Jenner and his great contribution to mankind. Napoleon respected Jenner because he gave his knowledge and vaccine free to all, friends and foes alike.

Nancy, France 1801: Napoleon and Josephine's carriage came to a halt in the city of Nancy for a change of horses and to allow the couple to refresh themselves. An Englishman, a Mr. Williams, was part of the multitude that had assembled to see and pay homage to their Emperor and his beautiful but inscrutable and unfaithful wife, Josephine. Hoping to attract the Emperor's attention, Mr. Williams waved an envelope in the air, but Napoleon ignored the gesture. Williams then added his voice to the visual signal and sang out at the top of his voice, "Jenner, Jenner." Still, Williams' entreaties went unnoticed, so he pushed himself forward into the gathering to get closer to Napoleon, but as luck would have it, he was restrained by the guards. But luck is a fickle and seductive mistress, who comes and goes as she pleases; she can be neither bought nor sold; and whosoever she chooses to be with, the choice always is hers.

Napoleon, for all his military genius and meticulous planning before a battle, was still a great believer in luck. It would seem that, if an unexpected event happened during a battle, it always seemed to favor him. If it rained without warning, it was his enemy's gun powder that got wet and made useless, never his. Whenever Napoleon selected a new general, no matter how well qualified the man, the last question he asked his staff was "But is he lucky?" The question Napoleon was asking his staff was: no matter how carefully and intelligently this general planned his battles, would "Mistress Luck" favor him and not his enemy?

But this day, luck was with Mr. Williams, because Josephine heard his voice calling out the name, "Jenner." Reaching out, Josephine touched Napoleon's arm to gain his attention, saying, "Sire, that man waving a piece of paper cries out the name, Jenner."

Napoleon instructed a guard to immediately bring the man holding the paper to him. The guard quickly forced his way through the congestion, and gaining access to the man with the paper, notified him that the Emperor wished to see him. Williams, holding on to the back of the soldier's thick-leather waist-belt, was pulled through the crowd and presented to Napoleon.

Napoleon turned and remarked to Josephine, "Jenner! Ah, I wonder what this man wants. I am beholden to Dr. Jenner for giving the world vaccination. How can I ever refuse that saintly and unselfish man anything?"

Napoleon, more than anyone else in Europe, gave recognition to the fact that by freely giving his discovery of cowpox vaccination, Jenner had made a major contribution to all mankind. France, more than any other nation, benefited the most from Jenner's discovery. Jenner had supplied French doctors with cowpox vaccine to be used for vaccinating the French population. Napoleon, ever alert to new discoveries, especially those that had military value, sent two of his military doctors to visit Jenner to learn how to properly administer the vaccine. When England and France were at war with each other, both Napoleon and Wellington had their armies vaccinated.

Mr. Williams handed Jenner's letter to Napoleon, which he carefully read.

"Sire,

Having by the blessing of Providence, made a discovery of which all nations acknowledge the beneficial effects, I presume upon that plea alone, with great deference, to request a favour from your Imperial Majesty, who early appreciated the importance of vaccination, and encouraged its propagation, and who is universally admitted to be a patron of the arts.

My humble request is that your Imperial Majesty will graciously permit two of my friends, both men of science and literature, to return to England; one Mr. William Thomas Williams, residing in Nancy; the other Dr. Wickham, at present in Geneva. Should your Imperial Majesty be pleased to listen to the prayer of my petition, you will impress my mind with sentiments never to be effaced.

I have the honour to be with most profound deference and respect, Your Imperial Majesty's most obedient and humble servant,

Edward Jenner"

Napoleon acknowledged Jenner's request and, eventually, both men were released and permitted to return to England. What is so unusual about this incident is that, during a time of war between England and France, Jenner was able to arrange to have English prisoners released by the good graces of the Emperor Napoleon; moreover, Napoleon later had a medal struck in honor of Jenner and his discovery. It is without parallel that, during wartime, the ruler of one country honors a person who is a subject of his enemy.

Without a doubt, Napoleon's action of honoring Jenner with a medal during wartime was extraordinary, but Napoleon was no ordinary general. Napoleon knew, without question, that he was superior to any general in England or, for the matter, Europe; however, there was one enemy he couldn't defeat and that was smallpox. If a smallpox epidemic should occur in his army, at a critical time, disrupting its ability to fight, Napoleon would be helpless in the face of his enemies. Jenner's vaccination removed that threat, and, for that, Napoleon was eternally grateful.

Fierce sea battles were fought between England and France: The Battle of the Nile and the clash of the two giants, off the Spanish coast overlooking the headlands of the Cape of Trafalgar—the site where Horatio Nelson gained his greatest victory over Napoleon—brought with it everlasting fame and glory for Nelson.

The spread of vaccination throughout Europe could have been hampered during the war, except that Britain controlled the channel separating England and France. This permitted correspondence between England and Europe to continue in an orderly fashion, enabling Jenner to send his vaccine to most European countries, during the most turbulent of times.

Napoleon too, without realizing it, enabled Jenner's vaccine to be distributed safely throughout Europe. During Napoleon's conquest of much of Europe, order was maintained and the civil services continued to be well organized, including the mail; hence, Jenner was able to send his vaccine throughout Europe, even when England and France were at war with each other.

In 1801, a Dr. Aubert was sent by Napoleon to see Jenner in London for the purpose of obtaining information about vaccination. The doctor planned on establishing the first Vaccination Institute of France which was to be located in Paris. When Dr. Aubert returned to France, public vaccination became a national priority, but only after the soldiers of Napoleon's French Imperial Army had been vaccinated.

Was it any wonder then that Jenner should be acclaimed the man who saved the world? Still, life has its many little tricks to play on us, and even such a modest and successful man as Jenner could not manage to go through life without confronting life's many little foibles and pitfalls.

22

"JENNER NOT ONLY DISCOVERED VACCINATION, but he forecast what the future would be like, after vaccine was used worldwide." The Prof continued, "If Jenner had our knowledge that a virus, a living organism, caused smallpox, he would have more correctly said that the smallpox virus could no longer exist, if everyone were immune to the disease. It is the nature of the smallpox virus that humans are its only sanctuary. Jenner was correct, when he said that smallpox could be controlled worldwide by the use of his cowpox vaccine, even though it took another one-hundred-seventy years to demonstrate the correctness of his statement.

"But, like any good scientist, not all his predictions were correct. A case in point, Jenner published that vaccination caused permanent immunity against smallpox. This isn't true; the immunity lasts about ten years, but this wasn't determined for many years after Jenner published his *Inquiry*.

"During the Franco-Prussian War, Germany routinely revaccinated its troops, who were relatively free of smallpox during the entire war. France, on the other hand, refused to accept the need for revaccination, and as a result, the French troops suffered badly from the disease. Cattle-cars loaded with soldiers infected with smallpox had to be removed from combat and returned to Paris for medical care."

Ruth, having a resurgence of energy, after drinking a cup of stale, lukewarm coffee, spoke up, "Jenner never said anything about biological warfare using smallpox as a weapon, and the need for vaccination as the only protection."

"Of course, you are correct, Ruth. Jenner was too much of a humanitarian to even imagine such a thing," the Prof replied approvingly. "But truthfully and as you know well, biological warfare and bioterrorism, using smallpox, have been around for a long time, much before Jenner's discovery of vaccination. Even today, we are acutely conscious that smallpox could be used, once again, as a weapon. It is a subject that deserves mention, so suppose you inform us, Ruth." The Prof encouraged her to speak, which really wasn't necessary, since she loved to fascinate people with war stories, ever since the time she had been a soldier in the Israeli army.

"Fine, Prof, I'll do my best. The reason that I brought up the subject was that we tend to think of biological warfare, the use of a germ to produce disease in an enemy, as something relatively recent. But it is not. As you said, biological warfare dates back to the early sixteenth century and, perhaps, beyond. It is important to remember that smallpox was one of the first germs to be successfully employed as a weapon.

"Smallpox-infected garments were deliberately used, on many occasions, to purposefully cause the disease. The American Indians were the recipients of many biological attacks by smallpox. In 1763, Indian tribes successfully attacked Fort Pitt—which is the site of present day Pittsburgh—destroying British settlements outside the fort, because the fort was inadequately garrisoned to protect the area. The soldiers at the fort were frantic and smallpox was present among the troops. The British, in desperation, requested permission from the British high command to use smallpox as a weapon against the attacking Indian tribes. The answer to their request stated: 'We must, on this occasion, use every stratagem in our power to reduce them.' It was a typical British elliptical way of saying 'yes.' The officers in the fort then arranged to have smallpox-infected blankets fall into the hands of the hostile Indians. Eventually, an epidemic of smallpox developed among the attacking tribes and the encirclement of the fortification was broken.

"Smallpox was also used to kill off Indians from lands desired by white settlers. In 1752, during a smallpox epidemic, a letter was written saying, in effect, that 'It was desirable that smallpox should break out and spread generally throughout the localities inhabited by our Indians. Its use would be fully as good as an Army.'

"The early centuries in America are replete with examples of smallpox being used as a biological instrument of war and revenge. Various methods of spreading smallpox among the Indian tribes were used, but during the 17th century, blankets and handkerchiefs infected with crusts and pus, from patients with smallpox, seemed to be the common way the settlers spread the disease among the tribes. The American Indian tribes paid a huge price in deaths and disabilities, following the white man's colonization of the American continents. Far more Indians died of smallpox than were killed by the white man's bullets.

"Intentional use of smallpox as a biological weapon occurred during the Revolutionary War, when the English troops restricted to Boston were besieged by George Washington's army, located in the hills overlooking the city. Civilian refugees, intentionally infected with smallpox by the British, were forced to leave the city in hopes of infecting Washington's Continental army surrounding Boston. Fortunately, Washington was able to slow the spread of the disease by quarantining and disinfecting the refugees. When the British troops finally left Boston, Washington, as a precaution, ordered one thousand soldiers, known to have had smallpox, to occupy the city. Nevertheless, many of the soldiers and civilians in the city became seriously ill with smallpox."

Sarah quickly entered the conversation, "These were certainly cowardly events in the history of smallpox, and we all should be ashamed. But let's not forget that the threat of smallpox being used by terrorists is of paramount importance today. Prof, we should bring the subject of biological warfare and bioterrorism up-to-date and into the twenty-first century."

"Good idea, Sarah, and as long as you mentioned the subject, I wish that you would continue," was the Prof's reply.

"If you say so, Prof," Sarah responded. "With the knowledge of how the British successfully used smallpox as a biowarfare agent in the eighteenth century, interest in germ warfare developed in the military establishments of many countries. It wasn't until World War II, however, that the United States army seriously considered using smallpox as a biological weapon. It wasn't long before the research was discontinued, because the infectious nature of the smallpox virus could not be adequately controlled. The Japanese army, on the other hand, was able to develop an aerosol-spray containing smallpox, which they used successfully on Chinese prisoners in Manchuria. Other than that episode, the aerosol-spray was never used during WW II.

In the United States, in 1969, all biological warfare work was stopped, by order of the president. Actually, the smallpox virus was never judged to be an especially good agent for spreading disease. Furthermore, vaccination was considered an effective method of prevention, were it to be used as a military weapon. At the time, vaccination was still compulsory in the advanced countries of the world, so that the armies and the civilian populations were protected against the disease.

"Nevertheless, the Soviet Union, starting in 1928, developed a smallpox biological weapons program that was considerably ahead of all the western European nations, including the United States. By 1947, Soviet scientists considered the smallpox virus as the biological weapon of choice: it was strong enough to withstand an explosive delivery charge; very infectious when delivered through the air; could cause mass casualties and produce panic among both the army and civilian populations.

"For many years, Soviet scientists continued to search for a strain of smallpox virus most suitable for production as a weapon. By accident, in 1967, a strain of smallpox virus was isolated from an Indian tourist visiting Moscow. As a euphemism, the virus strain was given the secret code name of India-1. Eventually, India-1 proved to be an excellent virus strain for military purposes, and the virus was soon grown in massive amounts by inoculating the virus into the membranes of fertilized chicken eggs.

"Once adequate supplies of the virus were weaponized, warheads filled with the virus were mounted on intercontinental ballistic missiles, placed in silos close to the Arctic Circle, and were made ready to be launched on notice from the Kremlin.

"By 1972, world opinion forced the Soviet union to become a member of the Biological Weapons Convention, which drew up an international treaty banning disease agents and natural poisons as weapons of warfare. However, since 1969, the United States had voluntarily banned the use of these agents, and at the time, the Soviet Union also agreed, knowing full well that any violation of the agreement on their part would not be detected, since adequate inspections for violations were not possible.

"It was ironic that, in 1973, the Kremlin appointed Dr. Viktor M. Zhdanov, a highly respected virologist and a member of the elite Soviet Academy of Sciences, as head of the agency for the secret development of biological warfare agents. The sole purpose of this agency was to work on weaponization of the smallpox virus. It was the same Dr. Zhdanov who, as Deputy Minister of Health, had first suggested the global eradication of smallpox, in 1958, at the World Health Assembly meeting in Minneapolis. While the Soviet Union denied having weaponized smallpox, the military command had stockpiled twenty metric tons of it at their Center of Virology in the city of Zagorsk.

"As long as the masses of the Western world remained vaccinated, the threat of the Soviet stockpile of smallpox was limited to that of producing panic and only a moderate number of casualties. Therefore, compared with other weapons systems, such as atomic bombs and weaponized toxic gases, smallpox seemed to be of limited value. But, unexpectedly, 'Lady Luck' favored the Soviet military, and not her adversaries, for in 1980, the World Health Organization declared the global eradication of smallpox, something Jenner had predicted one-hundred-seventy years earlier. Now, the vaccination of the world's civilian populations was stopped. The Kremlin saw this as a military opportunity against the west, in particular the United States.

"Despite knowing that the Soviet population, itself, was also susceptible to being infected with their smallpox virus, the Kremlin, in 1980, ordered the discontinuance of vaccination of the Soviet people. If they would have done otherwise, it would have tipped their hand that they still intended to use the smallpox virus as a biological weapon.

"By 1985, the world situation had become so tense that the Soviet Union saw no need to vaccinate their own people, even if they were to use the smallpox virus as a weapon. The world crisis had evolved into a weaponry nightmare. The Soviets anticipated destroying their enemy by first using atomic bombs and then exposing those who survived to the smallpox virus.

"Frightening isn't it?" Sarah said, letting out a deep sigh.

"During the nineteen-eighties and early nineties, the Soviets continued to expand their secret programs to improve their weaponization of the smallpox virus. This included the production of a more contagious form of the disease. In an attempt to keep the program a secret, those working on the project were vaccinated on their buttocks, to avoid the telltale scar on the upper arm, the usual site for vaccinations. These workers were also kept in isolated towns, away from the general population. The smallpox weaponization project continued to expand and become more sophisticated in its methods of delivery. By now, the Soviet Union had planned on delivering bomblets filled with weaponized smallpox by their large, long-range TU-95 bombers, in addition to using their new intercontinental ballistic missiles, which were usually restricted for delivering atomic warheads. The Soviets relented and permitted some of their prized ballistic missiles to carry warheads containing their new, deadly, smallpox virus.

"As scientific research methods in gene identification and genetic engineering advanced, the Soviet Union began using these new procedures for their own purposes of making a more deadly form of the smallpox virus. Soviet scientists quickly directed their energies towards discovering the gene sequences of the smallpox virus and relating these genes to their function and mode of operation. Once this was accomplished, it was then possible to compare the smallpox genetic structure with the genetic structure of the other pock viruses, such as monkeypox and mousepox, to determine which genes produced infectivity and pathology in humans.

"Eventually, the Soviet genetic engineering program reached the stage where weapons-grade smallpox was to be up-graded, by transferring to the smallpox virus structure virulent genes from the Ebola hemorrhagic fever virus. Such a virus combination would take advantage of the infectivity of smallpox with the killing power of the Ebola, which was ninety to one hundred percent effective as a lethal weapon.

"Fortunately, a senior biological scientist, Dr. Vladimir Pasechnik, defected to the West, during a visit to France, and revealed the vast biological weapon programs involving the smallpox virus that the Soviet Union had been able to hide from the rest of the world.

"After the collapse of the Soviet Union, in 1991, all research involving the weaponization of the smallpox virus either was stopped or drastically reduced. As luck would have it, by then, the new genetically engineered strains of the smallpox virus were still not usable for biological warfare. Supposedly, seed cultures of smallpox virus were restricted to a repository in Moscow, but there was no assurance that terrorist states or organizations had not obtained samples of smallpox for their own diabolical purposes, or that rogue Soviet scientists had not left Russia to work for terrorists organizations."

"Thank you, Sarah," said Prof, "I think it is time that we return to our friend, Dr. Jenner. While he was in the midst of receiving accolades and awards from all over the world, at home in England, he still had many problems. Cedric, bring us up-to-date, please," the Prof concluded.

Cedric, as usual, was delighted to share his knowledge with the rest of the group. Modesty was not one of Cedric's strong points, as everyone knew.

"Well!" Cedric began, "As was the custom...."

◆ ◆ ◆

As was the custom of that time, it was to be expected that Jenner would receive a sinecure or a straightforward financial award from the King or the national treasury for his remarkable discovery. There were many examples of people receiving such awards for work that was of value to the crown or to the country. Some awards, however, were not so much meritorious as they were political. A person, such as, Dr. Samuel Johnson (1709–84), the lexicographer, rightfully earned a lifetime pension for producing his distinguished dictionary of the English language; while on the other hand, there were people like a Mr. Stephens who produced a solvent for stones—which in the end did not work—and was awarded 5,000 pounds.

In such situations "pulling strings," so to speak, was considered a guiltless sport, and it was conceded that any official in the government, who failed to look after his friends, was thought to be a bit of a scoundrel.

During ensuing debates in Parliament about an award for Jenner, there were few politicians to champion his cause, since, over the years he remained aloof from politicians and politics. Still, his discovery was of such great importance that, unknowingly, he had many friends and admirers in high places in government.

It was generally agreed, but unfortunately not by everyone, that the discovery of vaccination as a method of preventing smallpox was superior to the old method of variolation, introduced into the country by Lady Montagu, early in the eighteenth century.

Vaccination saved more lives and prevented more blindness, disfigurement and deformities than any other medical treatment, up until that time. The benefits to England, in lives saved alone, enabled the country to grow and become a wealthy and powerful nation. Justice would dictate that Jenner deserved a large award for his work, especially when it is recognized that he derived no financial benefit from his discovery. He personally paid all his own research expenses, and distributed the vaccine with personal handwritten instructions free to anyone worldwide requesting it. Moreover, he rarely charged a patient coming to him to be vaccinated. All seemed to agree, had any other doctor discovered vaccination, he would have become a rich man. Jenner, on the other hand, was not rich, but neither was he poor, for he had a small income from his wife's inheritance, and the income from his medical practice in Berkeley, which was rather meager.

The Earl and Countess of Berkeley organized a written campaign on behalf of their friend, Dr. Jenner. It was a start, but in order to win an award from Parliament, he needed many more friends to promote his cause.

Jenner was advised by his friends that, before he could obtain a grant from the government, he would have to write a petition and have it presented to Parliament by one of its members. The amount of work, on his part, would be extraordinary. There was the petition to be prepared; a speech to be written and presented before parliament; a visit with the Prime Minister and meetings with influential members of Parliament; as well as discussions with numerous dignitaries representing the crown. In addition, he was being overwhelmed with all manner of advice—some good, some bad. Altogether, it was not the type of social environment that Jenner enjoyed, and, at times, he became a bit impatient. Regardless of all the irritations, in the middle of December 1801, Jenner had to move to London to facilitate his petitioning the government for a grant.

Finally, after three months of tedious and boring preparations, a petition was presented in the House of Commons by a Mr. Mildmay on behalf of Dr. Jenner. The House was informed that both the King and the Prince of Wales approved and recommended the award. A committee was established, under the guidance of Admiral Berkeley, brother of the Earl of Berkeley, Jenner's friend and sponsor. It is of interest that Jenner's brother, the Reverend G. C. Jenner, attended these meeting and took notes, which he published at a later date.

Like all inquiries, much time was wasted on long drawn-out speeches, many unrelated to the topic under discussion. The committee was formed to answer three questions: "Were the effects of vaccination entirely beneficial?" "Was Dr. Jenner the discoverer of vaccination?" and "What pecuniary advantage or increase in practice had he reaped from it?"

One would think that the answers to such questions would have been easy, and the committee's work simple, realizing that the rest of the world was committed to honoring Jenner for his work. But, frequently, even simple things can be made complicated, and so they were at Jenner's hearing.

The Admiral, in order to move the hearing along, immediately proposed that an award of 10,000 pounds be made to Jenner. This was much less than he deserved, but the Admiral anticipated this, and in his remarks suggested that anyone wishing to increase the award could do so. The suggestion was received favorably.

"Were the effects of vaccination entirely beneficial?" This was the first question the committee asked. In the process of answering the question, Jenner was challenged by many doctors and surgeons who, quite obviously, did not approve of vaccination, but were also unqualified to discuss the subject. The cross-examination lasted for days, and, at one point in the relentless questioning, Jenner saw fit to write to a friend, complaining: "Having been put in possession of the laws of vaccination by so great a number of the first medical men of the world...they (the parliamentary committee) should not have listened to every blockhead who chose to send up a supposed case of its (vaccination's) imperfections; but this is the plan pursued, and if they (the committee) do not give up, they (the committee) may sit to the end of their lives (listening to worthless speeches)." The major objection to vaccination that these doctors and surgeons had hoped to make was that vaccination did not work.

Jenner was right to be upset. The leading specialists of the world examined the practice of vaccination and accepted Jenner to be the discoverer of one of the world's greatest contributions to medicine.

While many of the doctors and surgeons that came before the committee were disparaging about vaccination, yet, there were those distinguished individuals and doctors who spoke favorably about it. For instance, the Earl of Berkeley and the Duke of Clarence, the son of the King, both gave examples of the value of being vaccinated. Sir Walter Farquhar, physician to the Prince of Wales, added that: "I think it (vaccination) is the greatest discovery that has been made for many years." A surgeon, a Mr. Cline, came closer to the truth when he said: "It (vaccination) is the greatest discovery ever made in the practice of Physic (medicine) for the preservation of human life; as the smallpox has been more destructive than any other disease." A Dr. Heberden estimated: "that if vaccination were made compulsory, an average of ninety-three lives per day would be saved in the United Kingdom."

As the questioning by the committee progressed, even more lucid and knowledgeable doctors were questioned. Next to present was a Dr. Saunders, Senior Physician at the prestigious Guy's Hospital. He assured that from his experience, vaccination was both effective and safe to use. His final statement was both unequivocal and prescient when he said: "That it (vaccination) is one of the most important discoveries ever made for the benefit of the human race, and that if the practice continues and prevails, it (vaccination) bids fair ultimately to extirpate the poison (virus) of the natural (acquired) smallpox."

Even the chairman of the committee, Admiral Berkeley, who supposedly should have been neutral, took a deep breath, signifying his complete satisfaction, after listening to such a forthright statement, from such a distinguished physician, supporting vaccination and Jenner. A debate about the efficacy of vaccination, which began so poorly, ended up as a victory for Jenner.

The second question to be debated: "Was Dr. Jenner the discoverer of vaccination?" After Jenner published the *Inquiry,* and the success of vaccination became generally known and accepted, claims for priority were made by people in both England and Europe. The reports were of little scientific value, but they were used by some of Jenner's detractors as a means of discrediting him.

Initially, Jenner made no claim of priority of discovery when he published the *Inquiry*, but only did so later on, at the encouragement of his friends, to neutralize the claim by Dr. Pearson that he was the true originator of vaccination. This is the same nefarious Dr. Pearson of London who initially befriended Jenner, only to, later on, lay claim to the discovery of vaccination. As expected, it was a claim that no one in the scientific community took seriously.

Of all the claims of priority to vaccination, a farmer named Benjamin Jesty, deserves mentioning, since Jesty's name was frequently raised at the hearing. Jesty knew of the stories that having had cowpox would prevent a person from contracting smallpox. During the smallpox epidemic of 1774, Jesty learned that a neighbor's cows had the lesions of cowpox on their udders. With that information, Jesty decided to take his wife and two young sons to a field where the cows were grazing and removed some matter from the pustules on a cow's udder. Afterwards, he scratched the arms of his wife and two sons with a needle and deliberately rubbed the infectious material into the wounds. He had, in reality, vaccinated them. The inoculations were successful, since none of them developed smallpox, during the epidemic. The children had no reaction to the inoculation, but his wife, who initially nearly died of fever, later recovered. Once his neighbors learned what Jesty had done, he was treated as a pariah and, even though his wife recovered, he was called a murderer. The maltreatment did not end there. For the longest time, the villagers taunted him for being a witch, and they pelted him with mud and rocks. Jesty withstood the deluge of scorn but, once it was over, he never again was tempted to brag about his experiment. Nothing came of the Jesty episode, except that in 1805, he was given a testimonial and gold-mounted lancets by the Vaccine Pock Institution, of which the notorious Dr. Pearson was in charge.

Unsuccessful charges were made by Jenner's detractors that he had known of these earlier attempts at vaccination. It is difficult to know all that is going on, even in this day of rapid communications; during the eighteenth century, it must have been nigh impossible. The committee's conclusions were simple. In all the priority claims made at the committee hearing, none of them were made before Jenner's *Inquiry* was published in 1798, and none influenced how doctors prevented smallpox. Jenner was the first and only person to scientifically test and evaluate vaccination as a means of preventing a smallpox infection in an individual and, afterwards, make his findings known to the worldwide medical community.

As much as Dr. Pearson tried to malign Jenner's reputation at the committee hearing, it was his own reputation that came under question before the sessions ended. It seems that Dr. Pearson made some misleading statements about vaccination and quoted the, by now, world famous Dr. Heberden. Heberden, by this time quite old and feeble, came out of his retirement to challenge the truthfulness of Dr. Pearson's statements. The evidence presented before the committee all favored the fact that Jenner was the rightful originator of vaccination. The committee decided to by-pass the question, "Was Jenner the first to discover vaccination?" and settled the issue on the unquestioned fact that he was the first to use person-to-person serial vaccinations.

But there were many other reasons for honoring him. He was the first one to identify true cowpox and knew how to preserve the active vaccine. He was also the first to identify a true vaccine pustule, after a person had been vaccinated. And he had spent many years of his time and much of his fortune convincing the medical world to use vaccination for the good of all mankind.

The third and final question to be taken up was: "What pecuniary advantage or increase in practice had Jenner reaped from the discovery of vaccination?" As the committee quickly realized, the answer to the question was he did not receive any financial gain from his discovery. A committee member pointed out that it was more correct to asked, "What had he lost?" The committee member then attempted to answer his own question and replied, "He has actually lost the opportunity of making his fortune, by making it (vaccination) public." One member said that he could have made ten thousand pounds a year, which was an astronomical figure for the time. Still another said the amount should be twenty-thousand pounds a year, and yet another put the number more dramatically by asserting: "I think he might have died the richest man in all the dominions."

The problem next arose how to put a monetary value on all the lives that Jenner saved with the use of vaccination. One statistically minded member concluded that forty thousand lives were saved yearly in the United Kingdom, with each life worth the paltry sum of ten shillings, an almost laughable amount. Still, even at that rate, Dr. Jenner would be entitled to twenty thousand pounds yearly.

There were other members of the committee who were jealous of Jenner's achievements and wanted to award him a trifling six hundred pounds. Finally, with some outside pressure from the Prime Minister, who was intent on keeping an eye on the budget while, at the same time, concerned about a war with France, the amount settled was ten thousand pounds. Not much of an award, when Jenner's expenses associated with preparing for the award, amounted to six thousand pounds.

In 1806, Parliament, realizing they had made a grievous mistake in their treatment of Jenner, agreed to correct the mistake by awarding him a further sum of twenty thousand pounds. Nevertheless, the opinion of most members of the awarding committee was, despite these grants, Jenner was financially the loser, as a result of his monetary obligations to advance the cause of vaccination and to supply vaccine, without charge, to anyone in the world requesting it from him.

23

"DURING OUR DISCOURSE, THERE HAVE BEEN comments made about the global eradication of smallpox infection, which, by the way, was one of Jenner's expectations for vaccination," the Prof remarked, wishing to move the discussions along, but not wanting to leave out any important detail.

Since the global eradication program eventually came to be directed by an American doctor, Jimmy assumed the prerogative of starting the discussion. "Prof, let me get things started, since I knew some of the people, personally, who were involved in the program."

The Prof was only too delighted to have such an alert and attentive volunteer. "Excellent, Jimmy, tell us what you know."

"The idea of global eradication of smallpox had been around a long time, and as we have frequently mentioned, it was first suggested by Jenner at the very end of the eighteenth century. The idea was not seriously considered as realistic, until it was offered as a proposal by Dr. Victor Zhdanov of the Soviet Ministry of Health, at a United Nations assembly meeting in Minneapolis, Minnesota, in 1958.

"Zhdanov was an intellectual who could just as easily quote from the framers of the American Constitution as he could from Lenin or Marx. He was equally learned in virology and public health matters, so he had to be taken seriously. In addition, he had the backing of the, then, powerful Soviet Union. His proposal amounted to a typical Russian five-year-plan. During the first two years, all countries would produce and stockpile cowpox vaccine, and in the remaining three years, there was to be a world population vaccination campaign against smallpox.

"Zhdanov reasoned that, since smallpox was a disease restricted to humans without any animal or insect host, it could be eradicated by making sure that everyone in the world was properly vaccinated. While this sounded like a formidable task, and it actually was, still in Europe and North America, most of the people had already been vaccinated and smallpox was absent from these countries.

"Total vaccination of the world population was an accepted idea for eradicating certain infectious diseases, including smallpox, but there are problems with this concept, which we shall see later. But I am getting ahead of myself, so, once again, let me backtrack a bit.

"The World Heath Organization, better known by the initials WHO, is an arm of the United Nations, and was founded in 1948, with headquarters in Geneva, Switzerland. WHO was a reluctant sponsor of the smallpox global eradication program, since it was already sponsoring its own programs of attempting to eradicate malaria and measles. They feared that starting another program, such as smallpox, would divert attention away from their malaria and measles programs which were receiving good financial support.

"Still, despite many obstacles and pitfalls, the smallpox program got started, mainly through the political pressure exerted by the then dominant Soviet Union. Within a few years, however, the program was well on its way to becoming a failure. There were multiple reasons, such as, bureaucratic bickering, lack of proper funding and poor leadership.

"The Soviets lived up to their obligation of producing massive amounts of vaccine for the project. They were not directly involved, however, with the operation and administration of the program and, therefore, they were not responsible for its failure. But because they initiated the program and supported it with their cowpox vaccine, they were distressed with what was happening. The United States, on the other hand, gave minimal assistance to the program by sending a small unit of their CDC (Communicable Disease Center) to Africa, but the CDC was not in any way, at this time, responsible for the success or failure of the program.

"Before the program ended in complete failure, the United States assumed a leadership role, with the approval and support of the Soviet

Union. This was important, since politically the two countries were at odds with each other. The United States assumed its new job reluctantly, after having to put up with much bickering and international intrigue. The WHO and other countries schemed to promote their own best interests, and since there was no great enthusiasm for the program at the top administrative level of WHO, they were satisfied to relinquish the leadership position to the United States, with the idea that, if the program were to fail—as many expected it would—then it was a failure for the United States and not WHO. The fact that the eradication program was eventually a success almost contradicts all known administrative and scientific laws, and hence indirectly must have had some supernatural power supporting it.

"While the history of the global smallpox eradication program is a long and remarkably interesting story, I'll speed things up by only mentioning some of its more salient features. After the initial failure of the program, many countries, most importantly the United States and the Soviet Union, realized the total eradication of smallpox was necessary; and with their coaxing, the World Health Assembly voted for a new, intensified smallpox program which had, as its final goal, the elimination of smallpox from the planet, within ten years. The amendment was passed by a mere two votes, the closest voting margin in the history of the organization.

"The director general of WHO, the sponsoring organization, was certain that the eradication program would fail, damaging the reputation of his organization, even though it had the cooperation and backing of the United States and the Soviet Union. He called Washington and insisted that an American doctor be put in charge of the program, so that the United States would be blamed when the program failed—and not his organization.

"In 1966, a well trained, intelligent young doctor, by the name of Donald Ainslie Henderson, was put in charge of the smallpox eradication program. To say that he was happy about the appointment would be a mistake, for he knew that he was stepping into a quagmire of intrigue, conspiracies and intergovernmental collusions.

"Nevertheless, Henderson was a good choice to lead the program, since he was familiar with all the different agencies involved, and he knew the leaders and their idiosyncrasies. Most importantly, he demanded and received proper funding for the program; he developed an excellent, qualified and ambitious group of people to carry out the laborious work involved, and, finally, he had the support and loyalty of the scientists in the Soviet Union.

"As the eradication programs progressed in various countries, they were aided by dedicated workers responsible for finding and vaccinating large groups of people; in spite of this, it soon became evident that there were problems in the underlying strategy of the program that, eventually, would lead to its failure.

"Henderson was fortunate, though. Call it what you want—luck, destiny, karma—whatever it was, Henderson had it. At a crucial point in the program, it was discovered that there was something very wrong, and Henderson proved to be the right person to fix it.

"Thousands of workers were vaccinating millions of people, and while smallpox was being controlled in some areas, in other areas the program was a failure. This was particularly true on the Indian subcontinent where the fieldworkers were not making any progress with the disease, no matter how hard they tried. It was estimated that as much as eighty percent of the population had been vaccinated, but still the number of new cases rose.

"The idea that the total population needed to be vaccinated, in order for the program to be successful, was a firmly fixed theorem within the scientific community. The goal, then, was for the fieldworkers to vaccinate one hundred percent of the population. By the time eighty percent of the population was vaccinated some real progress was expected, but new cases were occurring at a higher rate than anticipated.

"The first bit of luck occurred in Nigeria, where there was an epidemic of smallpox. At the time there was a shortage of both vaccine and personnel, so the director of the area, Dr. William Foege, gave orders that when smallpox occurred in an insolated area, his staff was to stop their usual procedure of vacccinating everyone in that area, and instead concentrate on vaccinating only those individuals that had been exposed to the smallpox. Using this new approach, the smallpox epidemic was stopped and the disease was totally under control, within three short weeks.

"What Foege demonstrated was that it wasn't necessary to vaccinate everyone to control an epidemic of smallpox, as long as the persons with the disease were isolated and their immediate contacts vaccinated. By following this procedure, only a small number of people had to be vaccinated, in an area where new cases of smallpox occurred; and the disease could be quickly controlled and prevented from spreading to other towns or villages within the country. Foege and his staff had serendipitously stumbled onto something new and radical, without immediately grasping its full potential.

"It wasn't long, though, before Foege realized what had occurred and understood that the process had the potential for much wider application, perhaps to an entire subcontinent such as India.

"What Foege had previously been led to believe about smallpox wasn't necessarily correct—that an entire population had to be vaccinated for the smallpox virus to be eliminated. Foege learned, from experience, that smallpox consisted of small isolated areas of infection and that the virus moved about slowly, from person to person, never infecting everyone in an area at the same time. It was this characteristic of the smallpox virus that made it easy to isolate and prevent from spreading. The difficulty was in the identification of new cases of smallpox and their isolation. Following this, it was necessary to quickly find and vaccinate all the contacts of the new cases of smallpox. This was quite different from what he had expected. For example, when the smallpox season in West Africa occurred, the disease could be present in as few as one percent of the villages at any one time; and if the disease was immediately brought under control in those villages, the smallpox virus could be eliminated, and consequently, not spread to other parts of the country. Later, studies in India confirmed these same observations.

"The plan now changed from total population vaccinations to establishing a surveillance system that alerted the vaccinators where smallpox was occurring. Foege was also able to show where and when outbreaks of smallpox took place in eastern Nigeria. For instance, there was very little smallpox in eastern Nigeria, during the late summer and autumn seasons. The smallpox virus showed a similar occurrence in other countries, such as Pakistan, where smallpox was related to the monsoon season; smallpox occurred in the spring, preceding the heavy rains.

"Armed with this new knowledge, mass vaccinations were done during the season when smallpox was least likely to be present in the area. In Nigeria, for example, performing mass vaccinations during the autumn, when smallpox was least likely to be present, permitted the vaccinators to eliminate smallpox in Nigeria, in a period of five months. Besides, out of a total population of twelve million people, seven hundred and fifty thousand people had been vaccinated—a mere six percent of the population—which brought the disease under control.

"When the success in Nigeria became known, epidemiologists decided to use the experiment in eight other countries, and within a year, smallpox was eradicated from all these countries. The system consisted of dependable surveillance, that is, quickly identifying a smallpox outbreak; and using containment to stop the spread of the disease, by vaccinating the entire population where the disease was found. The war cry, for the vaccinators, now was "surveillance and containment."

"The practice of surveillance and containment varied slightly from country to country, but, in general, it produced good results in the laborious battle to eradicate smallpox. Before the smallpox virus was finally eradicated, there were still numerous interagency political and turf battles to be won, but Henderson proved to be the ideal person to meet these challenges. Finally, on October 26, 1977 a young man in Somalia, presented himself to the eradicator team with a rash which they diagnosed as smallpox. The man survived the disease and attained the dubious honor of being the planet's last case of naturally occurring smallpox."

"Excellent presentation, Jimmy. All those brave young men and women, representing so many different countries throughout the world, caused this event to happen and they deserve our heartfelt thanks," the Prof conceded. "We still have a way to go, before we are finished with the Jenner story, and I know, dear," addressing his wife, Iris, "that you have been following the story carefully and can continue from where we last left off."

Iris was delighted that Prof had invited her to speak again. She was beginning to feel left out of the discussions. And, of course, she knew what came next in the Jenner life story, for she was, after all, a medical doctor and could empathize with Jenner, for all the trials and tribulations he had faced proving to the world the value of vaccination for preventing the killer, smallpox.

"The years of hard work and long hours were beginning to show...."

◆ ◆ ◆

The years of hard work and long hours were beginning to show on Jenner, as he approached his 60th birthday in May of 1809. It was a time when he not only looked old but also had the physical sensations of being old. Worst of all, he could no longer keep pace with the extensive international requests for his vaccine, and for the first time, he required help to keep up with his voluminous correspondence and requests for vaccine.

The winter of '09 had been harsh, cruel and unforgiving, as only an English country winter can be. At the Chantry House in Berkeley, the passageways were especially cold and drafty, while the sitting rooms and bedrooms were only a trifle less so. Even though all the main rooms had fireplaces, they afforded the occupants little or no warmth. Indoors, both the family and the staff were required to wear warm clothing, and to dress much as they did when they were out-of-doors.

Inflammation of the joints, arthritis, was a common ailment. It came on during middle age and gradually became worse, as the years passed. Because of the continuous exposure to the dampness and extreme cold, whether inside the houses or outside, the English were also plagued with chilblains, a condition affecting the skin of the lower legs and feet and, at times, the hands and the ears. The color of the skin turned anywhere from pale pink to blood-red, while at the same time, maddening sensations of itching, burning and pain combined to torment the infected areas. In the worst cases, blistering, ulcerations and infections were also present.

During the decade after 1798, when the *Inquiry* was printed, Jenner's emotions seemed to fluctuate between extreme joy and marked depression, depending upon how vaccination was being received, and whether he was being extolled or impugned for his discovery.

It was during these years that, on two occasions, he was seriously ill with typhus and expected to die. After each illness, lengthy and laborious recoveries followed. Jenner knew that he had lived well past his life expectancy, for death came early to most people in those days. Many of his friends, relatives and family were already dead or were soon to die. Jenner was neither looking forward to death, nor was he afraid of it, since he was a religious man who believed in God and the hereafter.

There were times though, depression was caused not by the realization of growing old, but because he was unable meet his numerous responsibilities. For instance, he no longer was able to maintain his ongoing vaccination research and, at the same time, take care of his patients in both Berkeley and Cheltenham. His prodigious personal correspondence was an enormous drain on him. Most of all, though, it was the helpless feeling that came over him knowing that there was no cure for Catharine, his wife, who was slowly dying of tuberculosis of the lungs.

For years, Catharine had worried about her husband's health, while, at the same time, she, herself, was suffering from a serious pulmonary disease. Eventually Catharine's health completely deteriorated, but long before her death, she was confined to her own bedroom, where Jenner personally administered to her with tenderness and dedication. He arranged everything from overseeing to her comfort to supervising her medicines and special diet. He did these things gracefully and out of love. His gestures showed the affection and the complete devotion Jenner developed for his wife over the years of their long and happy marriage.

It was during Catharine's confinement that Jenner began dissociating himself from most of his friends and refused to attend social gatherings, if only to be near her if she needed him.

Nevertheless, there were happy times that Catharine could still share with her husband, for in the twilight of his life, recognition and honors were bestowed on Jenner in abundance. Vaccination had been universally approved as the preventative for smallpox in most countries and variolation was finally being banned worldwide. In spite of such universal acclaim, Jenner still had his detractors, who were mainly in London, where the erstwhile smallpox inoculators continued their archaic practice of variolation, until the mid-eighteen forties. Socrates, one of the most learned of Greek philosophers in the ancient world, was also denied by his countrymen, while being hailed by the rest of the civilized world. What a horrible loss to humanity, when impoverished Socrates was forced to commit suicide by his Greek countrymen, for having intellectual abilities and foresight much in advance of other men, mainly the politicians. Perhaps the biblical verse is correct, when it tells us that a prophet is least respected in his own homeland.

Now, almost totally confined of his home, Jenner remained immersed, as best he could, in his immense worldwide correspondence related to vaccination. Doctors, particularly in Europe and North America, were totally dependent upon him for guidance in the proper manner of vaccinating their patients, and for providing them with the precious cowpox vaccine. While much of the time England was at war with either France or the United States, the mail service continued, since the English navy controlled the seas and, as a consequence, English and friendly foreign vessels continued to transport their cargos, along with mail, around the world.

Letter writing wasn't the only way that Jenner was able to keep his creative mind engaged, during his extended period of isolation. Without planning or forethought, he returned instinctively to doing those things that he learned as a young man, since the aging brain seems best able to recall rather than learn something new. He reverted to the study of geology and comparative anatomy, but the subject that he enjoyed the most and which occupied much of his time was that of the migration of birds. It was a subject that would engage him, until the day he died.

It was during his time of seclusion that numerous doctors and scientists visited him, either to offer him solace or engage him in scientific discussions. Sir Humphry Davy, one of the leading English scientific experimenters of his time, was one of his most frequent visitors. Davy, among his numerous scientific inventions, was identified with the miner's safety-lamp which bears his name. While the two men often disagreed, still, they were intellectual equals, and their many evenings together satisfied Jenner's need to stay attuned to the outside world of science.

It was during one of his periods of depression that he received notice that the National Institute of France was bestowing upon him the coveted honor of Foreign Associate, in recognition of his discovery of vaccination. And there was more. He received, with great personal satisfaction, notification that The University of Oxford was awarding him an honorary Doctor of Medicine degree. Of all the hundreds of awards and honors that he received in his lifetime, this one gave him the most gratification, because, for financial reasons, he was the only Jenner in many generations who had not attended Oxford. Vaccination accomplished what poverty had prevented. Even more fulfilling was the fact that there was unanimous approval for awarding him the honorary degree, for such unanimity rarely occurred at Oxford.

Dr. Baron, his young colleague, accompanied him to Oxford for the ceremony. It was Baron who revealed to him that Oxford had been planning this move since 1798, shortly after the *Inquiry* was published, but they thought it advisable to wait until additional information became available in support of his claims for vaccination.

Jenner, by this time, had been esteemed by nearly all the learned societies in the world, except England's own Royal College of Physicians; that niggardly organization denied him recognition since, years before, he refused to take their mandatory test in Latin, a subject that he studied as a young schoolboy, but was less prepared to deal with in his old age. To nullify the Royal College's extraordinary behavior, Baron, who so admired Jenner, pointed out to him that genius is its own reward—a philosophic position which, perhaps, was more satisfying to Baron than to Jenner. It was the same Dr. Baron who, after Jenner died, became his biographer, producing a two-volume tome of his life and writings.

By chance, Jenner had heard of the plight of James Phipps who as a boy of eight, in 1796, he had injected with cowpox serum, from a pustule on the hand of an infected dairymaid, hoping to render him immune to smallpox. Later, the boy was variolated—inoculated with smallpox—and shown to be immune to the disease. Phipps was critical in proving Jenner's thesis that cowpox vaccination was a safe and effective deterrent against smallpox. But now, these many years later, poor Phipps was living in the most miserable of circumstances, desperately ill with the dreaded scourge, tuberculosis of the lungs, the same disease that had plagued Catharine, Jenner's wife, most of her adult life. Jenner moved Phipps into a little cottage that he had built for him behind his home in Berkeley. Jenner cared for poor Phipps the remainder of his life, which, unfortunately, was very short.

Finally, Jenner's beloved Catharine, who was constantly in his thoughts, began spitting up blood, an undeniable sign of advanced tuberculosis of the lungs. The symptoms of the disease were etched indelibly in Jenner's mind, for in London, at that time, one of six persons in the population died of the disease. Jenner elected to forsake living in London or Cheltenham and returned to the clean and invigorating air of Berkeley. Chantry Cottage, despite its damp and chilly rooms, had been their first home, so Jenner hoped that its sentimental value would have a beneficial effect on his dear Catharine. As much as Jenner tried to put the thought out of his mind, he was too good a doctor not to know that Catharine's time on this earth was ending.

At times, Catharine seemed to grow stronger, especially when the weather was warm and the sun was shining, but such periods were transient. Finally, she developed bronchitis, a curse to anyone with chronic lung disease, and for her it was the beginning of the end. Already debilitated from years of coughing and loss of blood, she no longer had the strength to carry on, and it was expected that she soon would die.

Jenner and Dr. Baron provided her with the best of care, but Catharine realized that such matters of life and death are, at times, out of the hands of man and solely at the beckoning of God. She was mindful that she was soon to die, but she had no fear. Baron attended her the night before she died, and was faced with a scene that he never forgot. Catharine was totally prepared to die and was completely ready to meet her Maker. She was surrounded by family and a few friends who seemed to glow in the light reflecting from her goodness. A righteous person was dying, and all present knew it. Catharine died peacefully on the 14th of September 1815, at the age of fifty-four years. Jenner was now sixty-six and they had been married 27 years.

Frequently the death of a much loved one is more difficult to resign oneself to than the contemplation of one's own death, and so it was with Jenner. He never recovered from this ultimate of conclusions. Catharine was buried in a vault in the Berkeley church alongside generations of Jenners. Jenner never really regained his health or composure after Catharine died. For a while, it seemed as if he could not wait until he was united with her in the grave. For the next two years, he secluded himself in his cottage, neglecting his medical practice, which fortunately was being covered by his two assistants. He was able to respond, at times, to the pledges and promises that he had previously made to further the cause of vaccination.

Jenner would have remained withdrawn in his Berkeley cottage, had it not been for his earlier appointment as Berkeley Magistrate, which required him to participate in a trial of the killing of a local gamekeeper by a group of farmers that had been poaching. In a conflict between the gamekeepers and the farmers, a fight ensued in which one of the farmers fired a shot that killed the gamekeeper. The trial was very distressful for Jenner, for while he knew that there were extenuating circumstances to account for the death, the law demanded that the farmer be executed.

The prolonged trial had been conducted in Cheltenham, and when it was over, Jenner was looking forward to returning to the solitude of Berkeley, only to find, when he returned there, that vaccination was again under attack. A new epidemic of smallpox had inundated England, and eventually reached proportions that made it one of the worst epidemics of the 19th century. The west of England had been overwhelmed by the disease, including the county of Gloucester where Jenner lived. London was also ravaged, causing the populace and many of the doctors to question the value of vaccination and reflecting badly on Jenner.

What the epidemic finally demonstrated was that towns, such as Cheltenham and Berkeley where Jenner had been in charge of the vaccination programs, were almost entirely free of smallpox. In cities such as London, however, where many of the doctors objected to mass vaccinations, or where vaccinations were either improperly performed, or the cowpox serum not suitably collected and stored, the occurrence of the disease was inordinately high. What began as a rejection of Jenner and vaccination ended up being a vindication of both.

By 1822, the Smallpox Hospital of London had finally adopted vaccination as the sole treatment for preventing smallpox, at last forsaking the practice of the outdated and dangerous variolation. By now the medical profession of London had also renounced variolation and had totally accepted vaccination as the method of choice for preventing smallpox. It was a long hard fight, which Jenner and his cherished vaccination finally won, for the benefit of all mankind. But it wasn't until years later, well after Jenner had died, that the Vaccination Act made Jenner's discovery, vaccination, the law of the land.

The vicissitudes of life, along with aging and chronic illnesses, were exacting their toll on Jenner. He had neither the energy nor the will to champion the cause of vaccination any longer. Finally, vaccination would have to meet the challenges and succeed without its progenitor. Luckily, by this time, vaccination had passed the test of time and could succeed on its own. When Jenner dropped the baton, there were many other doctors ready to pick it up and carry it to its logical conclusion, namely, the total elimination of smallpox from the planet earth.

Jenner, by chance, had been in Cheltenham when it was announced that the Duke of Wellington was scheduled for a return visit to the city. With the defeat of Napoleon, the Duke was now the most respected man in Europe, and upon his arrival in Cheltenham, there was a triumphant celebration. The Duke had expected to meet with Jenner. The Iron Duke could have helped the cause of vaccination at a most critical time. Vaccination had played a part in the Duke's victory by protecting his soldiers from the dreaded smallpox, at a time when every man was needed on the battlefield. Jenner, however, decided to leave Cheltenham for Berkeley, without visiting the Duke, thereby missing a golden opportunity to enhance the arguments favoring vaccination.

In the history of medicine, perhaps no other doctor knew as many world leaders, without using them for his own benefit, as did Jenner. It was a lost opportunity for Jenner not to visit with the Duke, but very much in the character of a man who refused to compromise his principles, which held that vaccination was his contribution to his fellowman and not a means to riches or self-gratification. So instead he left it up to his colleagues to talk with the Iron Duke about vaccination, which they did with great success, for the promulgation of the use of vaccination for preventing smallpox.

While Jenner may have been wearing down, the successes of vaccination were just beginning to grow. At a time when he was becoming physically less active, his daily correspondence from home and abroad continued to increase. In one exchange of letters, he was informed that during the past eight years, in the Kingdom of Denmark, there had not been a single case of smallpox, after vaccination was mandated in the country. These gratifying results were due to an edict by the King ordering the entire Danish population to be vaccinated. By now, Jenner was in his seventieth year, and while the news elated him, it failed to overcome the ravages of time that were slowly withering his body.

Jenner, more and more, became locked into his melancholy moods. He was being disturbed by the dreams of an aged old man, where the pleasing and disappointing events of one's past life are mixed in equal proportions. If he could forget only the unpleasant things, and recall only the things that he wished to remember, his sleep at night would be so much more restful. The closest that he could come to this ideal was when he was in Berkeley in the solitude he found near Catharine's grave.

While he was at peace with his thoughts of Catharine at Chantry Cottage, he was also slowly growing frail and weak until he collapsed in his garden and remained unconscious, for an extended period, until he finally regained consciousness and crawled into the house. Dr. Baron was notified and quickly responded. After examining Jenner, he realized that he had had a cerebral accident and had narrowly escaped death. Baron warned him that he had to slow down or his next attack could be fatal. But Jenner refused the advice and continued with his exhausting routine of letter writing. It was as if he were looking ahead to his death, in order to be reunited with his beloved Catharine.

Refusing to follow his doctor's directions that he slow down and let his body heal, Jenner was determined to complete the writing of a small booklet on vaccination, his last. Once he published the booklet, it failed to arouse much interest in England, since it did not cover any new information but, as usual, it was well received overseas.

By now, Jenner was a mere shell of his old self; he was chronically ill, weak, feverish and confined to his cottage in Berkeley. Having lost Catharine, he now was to suffer a different kind of loss. His only daughter, Catharine, who helped to sustain him after his wife died, was about to marry and move away. It was a great loss for Jenner who came to depend upon her for many things, just as he had depended upon his wife, Catharine. To hide his grief, over the loss of his daughter's leaving, he engaged in his letter writing with more zeal than ever before. He wrote to Baron, "In earlier days, indeed, at any period of my long life, I do not think there was ever a period when I worked harder. It is no bodily exertion, of course, that I allude to; but it is that which is far more oppressive, the toils of the mind."

The day before he died, he felt somewhat energized and ventured out to take a walk in the extreme cold of a January morning. It was a most unusual act since, by now, he rarely left the cottage, except on the warmest of days, to walk in his garden. This time out he wished to visit a small nearby community to make arrangements for fuel to be supplied to some poor people in the parish. His mission completed, on the way back, he visited one of his nephews who had a studio close by. When Jenner arrived the young man, who was in high spirits, was singing a Scottish tune. Jenner may have been feeble, but he never lost he ear for music, and detecting that his nephew was singing the wrong note was quick to correct him, and even sang a few stanzas himself. Since it was cold in the studio, Jenner went downstairs and brought back a pail of coal for the youth, at the same time jesting that the lad now had himself a man-servant. He returned to his cottage exhausted and went to bed early that night.

But time, the great arbiter of death, was about to grant Jenner his wish—to be with his wife, Catharine, in death. After arising the next morning, he soon collapsed into a coma, on the floor of the sitting room in his Berkeley cottage, on a bleak and frigid morning in 1823. A servant entered the sitting room, where Dr. Jenner took his breakfast, hoping to find him looking out the window at the garden that gave him so much pleasure. The servant heard a strange gurgling sound but, at first, he gave no notice to it and assumed it was water running off of the roof. Upon entering the room, he discovered that the doctor could not be seen sitting at his usual place on the couch, and before advancing farther, he called out to the doctor hoping to get his attention. When there was no answer, he hustled into the room and found the good doctor lying on the floor, unconscious, having a seizure. Obviously, he had fallen from the couch. Two years prior to this, the doctor had had a similar seizure, so this time the servant knew what was happening. Immediately, the doctor's two assistants, who were in the next room, were summoned.

There was now set in motion a series of urgent and extraordinary events to try to save the doctor's life. First, the trio carried the doctor to his bed, and dispatched a rider to Gloucester, some twenty miles away, to fetch Doctor Baron, Jenner's personal physician and one of his closest friends. In the meantime, the young doctors attempted to give assistance, as they waited for Baron's visit, but they were well aware that what was now happening to Dr. Jenner was different from his previous seizure; this time the end was at hand.

Only after Doctor Baron arrived was the diagnosis confirmed; Jenner had had a second attack of apoplexy, a stroke, but this time his condition was critical. He was unconscious; the right side of his body was paralyzed; the pupils of the eyes were reduced to pinholes, unresponsive to bright light; the breathing was noisy with intermittent periods when he stopped breathing altogether, followed by labored gasps for breath. Every effort was made to arouse him but to no avail. He had survived his previous stroke, but this time, his physical condition revealed that a large blood vessel was blocked on the left side, causing severe brain damage.

Baron, as a last desperate action, bled his patient, in hopes that would relieve the pressure on his brain. Beyond this heroic pretense, he had nothing to offer his friend and colleague. Baron sat at his patient's bedside exhausted, depressed and helpless. With his hands holding his head and his elbows resting on the chair-arms, Baron sat throughout the evening listening to the gasping breathing of his beloved friend. Doctor Baron refused food, drink or conversation and demanded to be left alone with his thoughts. Many times Baron had sat with patients while they died, but he was still able to face these experiences without a feeling of helplessness and despair. It was not so with his friend, Jenner. It was not an easy thing for Baron to watch Jenner die. Jenner remained in the never-never land, where he was neither living nor dead. Finally, at three o'clock in the morning of the 26th of January 1823, the venerable doctor died.

As the members of the household gathered around the bed and gazed steadily at the pale and lifeless body, the tears flowed freely, and from Baron could be heard a weeping and mournful intonation which sounded like, "May he go in peace. God rest his soul."

24

"WELL, WE ARE NEARING the end of our story, with the death of a truly great man," the Prof said in a profoundly sorrowful tone, and the hint of tears glistening in his eyes—one couldn't be sure. Staring straight ahead and looking pensive, he continued in the same sad and lamenting tone of voice, "The story we have painted sounds almost like one of the hallowed fairy tales of mankind. Still, can there be anything finer than a truth that appears totally unbelievable? There is always something stimulating about a man's supreme act, for, at times, such acts seem to rise above ordinary human capabilities; but it is by actions that man restores faith in himself and humanity."

"Thanks, Prof, that was lovely. We all appreciate hearing those words," Valerie said. "We agree with you that Jenner had all the characteristics of a great man."

The Prof followed up on Valerie's germane remark. "Ruskin expressed it best when he said: 'I believe that the test of a truly great person is humility. I do not mean by humility, doubts of his own ability, but great men have a curious feeling that greatness is not in them but through them, and they see something divine in every other man and are endlessly, foolishly and incredibly merciful.'

"Because he had these qualities, Jenner, in his crusade to do good, was at times vulnerable, stripped of the ability to protect himself from the darts and arrows directed at him by those who were less trustworthy and undeserving. Perhaps, if all of us followed in Jenner's footsteps, there would be less hostility and prejudice in the world.

"Now, for a somewhat more sobering topic, let us consider vaccination and terrorism. Murray, would you address this subject for us? And with this we shall bring to a close tonight's gathering."

"I'll do my best, Prof."

"The Russians abandoned their smallpox research program, as did the United States, and both countries put the last of their smallpox virus samples safely away in well guarded deep-freezers; and that was the end of the story of smallpox and the need for vaccinations. Jenner could at last rest peacefully, in his crypt next to his wife, and his life's ambition would now be complete. Or so everyone thought.

"The maliciously mischievous smallpox that killed 300 million people in the 20th century alone, and caused more human damage than any other infectious disease in history, was no longer available to torment mankind. Best of all, no one on this planet would ever again need to be vaccinated. The hallmark of vaccination was the tell-tale wrinkled and dimpled skin on the left forearm of males and the upper left thigh of females. These were the insignias that would soon lose their significance and quickly disappear.

"It was agreed that both countries, United States and Russia, would one day destroy their remaining smallpox cultures, but it did not happen that way. For political reasons, both countries procrastinated in destroying the smallpox cultures that they kept in deep-freezers. Regrettably, during this time, there were examples of laboratory technicians contracting smallpox and dying.

"Eventually, there occurred the terrifying events of 9/11 in New York City, when the World Trade Center towers were brought down by terrorists. Society decided that it needed ways of protecting itself from future terrorists' attacks. It was possible that the deadly smallpox virus was held by terrorists and could be used as a biological weapon, so the American government decided that the population needed to be vaccinated. It was now forty years since vaccination had been discontinued in the U.S. and the entire population was susceptible to the disease. There was some confusion and chaos mixed with fear in the country, then. It was as if the country had reverted to the time when Jenner first introduced vaccination to the world. Suddenly, there was an urgent need for huge quantities of cowpox vaccine, in order to vaccinate hundreds of millions of people against smallpox.

"What caused such a dramatic change in everyone's thinking was a report by bioterrorism experts that they suspected as many as nine countries were secretly stockpiling the smallpox virus to be used as a biological warfare weapon. Countries such as Iraq, Iran, Pakistan, North Korea, and others were all suspected of growing the smallpox virus for less than honorable reasons, even though they had previously proclaimed that they no longer possessed the virus.

"In the United States alone, it was determined that 500,000 health workers and 10 million emergency responders needed to be vaccinated immediately; and it was speculated that, perhaps, the entire population of the United States, over 250 million people, eventually would have to be vaccinated or revaccinated. Quite obviously, such tremendous quantities of vaccine were not available, nor could they be quickly produced, so the idea had to be shelved, temporarily.

"The plan that was decided upon was to set a priority system. Vaccinate only those people who needed to expose themselves in case of a smallpox attack. Such individuals were identified as emergency responders. Other individuals to be vaccinated were the health care workers in the hospitals who would be responsible for the care of patients who contracted smallpox. It all sounded so simple and easy in the beginning, but as soon as the plan was put into effect, there were problems, major problems.

"The Department of Health and Human Services initially promised to vaccinate about half a million doctors, nurses, and paramedics within 30 days. However, a mere 10,000 people agreed to be vaccinated or revaccinated. The remainder of the half million people outright refused vaccination, for a variety of reasons. But, fundamentally, people were afraid, because they knew that there could be serious side effects to the procedure. The risk of complications was rare but real. The vaccine was known to occasionally produce a generalized skin reaction that, if not treated properly and quickly, could lead to death. Another side effect was rare but debilitating when it occurred, and that was the destruction of brain tissue, that usually resulted in severe and permanent brain damage. Many of the health workers knew of these complications and, for this reason, feared being vaccinated or even revaccinated. The problem of vaccination was compounded even further, when some scientists, specializing in smallpox, couldn't agree on the proper course of action to follow when recommending a vaccination program. The main objection to vaccinating large numbers of people was that the complications of being vaccinated outweighed the risk of getting smallpox, during a biological terrorist attack. In addition, there were those who were concerned about financial compensation, if they developed a minor complication and could not return to work, for a period of time after being vaccinated. It would seem that the initial mass vaccination program was hastily conceived and poorly presented to the public.

"The government attempted to revitalize the mass vaccination program, by suggesting that a newer form of the smallpox vaccine caused only an infinitesimal chance of producing serious complications. As an example, the military showed that, when the new vaccine was given to a well screened, young military population of 450,000, there were fewer side effects, and no deaths attributed to heart or brain inflammation. Yet there were a few deaths of undetermined causes.

"In the general population, however, it was the older people with cardiac problems that could be at risk of cardiac complications and even death; therefore, it was recommended that that group of people should not be vaccinated. After the military information was presented to the public, most people felt that the new vaccine was still not absolutely safe, although they acknowledged that it caused fewer adverse reactions than the old 1972 vaccine.

"Later, there were complaints from nongovernmental scientists who pointed out that: You don't use, on a large number of people, a vaccine that could be lethal, in order to protect them against a disease that doesn't exist. They also pointed out that WHO declared smallpox eradicated in 1979, and there hasn't been a case of smallpox in the United State since 1977. But in the years before routine vaccination was stopped, in 1972, in the United States, the chances of contracting smallpox were greater, and, therefore, the argument for risking vaccination was stronger.

Yet, there were those who argued that there are some extremely dangerous people in the world who would like to kill Americans. Hence, it was the responsibility of the American government to protect its people, and it would be foolish for the government not to plan for the worse-case scenario. This same group of people pointed out that smallpox was still a very dangerous disease, and it could kill as many as one-third of the people who contracted it, during a bioterrorist attack.

"But for the present, while there was resistance on the part of health workers and early responders to being vaccinated, federal officials wisely advised that individual State Health Departments develop their own workable plans for detecting and coping with a smallpox attack by bioterrorists.

"In New York City, in 1939, some seamen were reported in the newspapers to have smallpox, and before they could be isolated and treated, they exposed an unknown number of people to the disease in that city. That incident caused a huge demand for vaccination by New Yorkers. Presently, it is anticipated that if smallpox, spread by terrorists, is ever detected in the American population, the demand for vaccinations and revaccinations will be so great that health systems will be overwhelmed; hopefully, the government has the foresight to stockpile adequate quantities of smallpox vaccine and, on short notice, can muster the necessary well-trained health workers who know how to use it properly."

"Murray, as complicated as things seem to be at the present, perhaps, they may become even worse in the future," Iris added to the conversation. "Today, we now know of individuals that we are identifying as 'superspreaders.' These individuals spew out deadly germs—as they speak, cough or sneeze—without themselves being seriously ill. Unfortunately, smallpox has its share of such superspreaders, and if one of them were to be let loose in the population, there could be big problems.

"Superspreaders have been known for a long time in medicine, and have been associated with such other diseases as typhoid fever, tuberculosis and staphylococcus infections. In the past, superspreaders have been labeled with descriptive titles such as, superinfectors, supershedders, and cloud cases, because of the invisible mist of infection that they leave trailing behind them.

"A present-day example of superspreaders is identified with the recently recognized SARS disease (severe acute respiratory syndrome) which began in China. A child there was such an extraordinary spreader of the disease, that the Chinese doctors nicknamed him 'the poison little emperor.' Then there was a Chinese doctor with SARS who, while at a dinner party in Hong Kong, infected 12 of the guests; afterwards, he flew on to Singapore, Vietnam and Canada, where he was able to infect still more people.

"But the classical case of a superspreader occurred in New York City, in 1907. The lady responsible for the spreading was known as 'Typhoid Mary.' Mary's real name was Mary Mallon. She was born in Ireland in 1869, and, after arriving in New York City, she cooked for some of the city's well-to-do families. After a while, Mary was caught by the New York City Health Department, since she spread typhoid disease in all of the families for whom she had been a cook. Undoubtedly, Mary knew she was carrying the disease, even though she herself was not sick, because when a doctor called on her for a stool sample, she threatened him with a carving knife. Eventually, it took five, big, Irish, New York City policemen to corner Mary and cart her off to a hospital where typhoid bacteria were found in her stool samples.

"Mary was quarantined but later released, although she still had typhoid bacteria in her stools. She promised the authorities that she would never again work as a cook. Mary was a sly one though; she changed her name to Brown and disappeared; however, she was found again, in 1915, working in a hospital, when there occurred a major epidemic of typhoid fever among the hospital patients. Mary, of course, was the hospital's cook.

"This time, the health department again quarantined her, and she remained quarantined for the next 23 years. In 1932, she had a stroke and was invalided. Interestingly, it was not long afterwards that penicillin was discovered at St. Mary's Hospital in London. Penicillin could have cured Mary, but she died, in 1938, before penicillin became available for use by the general public.

"Can you imagine what would happen if a terrorist organization let loose a small number of smallpox superspreaders throughout the western world? Besides, it is not beyond one's imagination that a terrorist group might develop a strain of the smallpox virus which could turn some people into superspreaders."

The Prof interrupted, coming to everyone's aid, when he said, "Please dear, let's not get too carried away with speculations. We have had a long, trying evening and some of the things you are saying are absolutely frightening."

"I'm sorry," Iris replied. "Let me reassure you that not everyone who contracts a disease can function as a superspreader. Superspreaders are special people, and why they spread a disease, without themselves becoming sick, is still unknown. There is speculation, however, that these people have some form of natural immunity that makes them resistant to the diseases they spread."

Valerie was quick to come to Iris' defense. "Iris is correct when she points out that there are still many dangerous individuals plotting ways to harm us." Valerie then changed the topic to the new monkeypox disease. "The United States recently had a scare that a new disease, monkeypox disease, which is biologically related to smallpox, might become prevalent in our country. Monkeypox virus belongs to the same family of pox viruses as the smallpox virus. Fortunately, cowpox vaccination will also protect a person against monkeypox disease. Good old Jenner came to our rescue again, 200 year later.

"Monkeypox was brought into the U.S. by six giant Gambian rats shipped into the country as pets from Ghana. The rats were carriers of the monkeypox virus. The monkeypox virus is a close relative of the smallpox virus, but it is less deadly and contagious. The disease causes a rash and fever. But, so far, no one has died of it. A major concern was that it would spread to other animals, such as dogs, cats and prairie dogs. These animals are all household pets and could pass on monkeypox to humans."

And of course Cedric would not let the subject rest, without interjecting one of his little distressing tidbits. "Things are now even worse than any one of you so far has mentioned," Cedric said, almost gloatingly. Recently a superbug has been genetically engineered, from a mousepox virus, that is capable of evading the cowpox virus used for vaccinating people. The new superbug, however, now only infects mice. It was genetically designed for experiments only. But can you conceive what would happen if a superbug form of smallpox could be produced by terrorists? It would mean that our present vaccination program would be useless against the new smallpox superbug, and all our discussion about national vaccination programs would be meaningless."

Sarah, more or less, spoke for the group when she said sarcastically, "Thank you, Cedric, I'm sure that after hearing your remarks, we will all sleep more soundly, knowing that such a horrible creature as a superbug could be growing in some terrible person's laboratory."

"Well we still have a little more of the Jenner story to tell before the evening is over, so perhaps Ruth will complete the story for us," the Prof said in a gentle tone, which he used when addressing a lady.

Ruth began by saying, "A concerted effort was made...."

◆ ◆ ◆

A concerted effort was made to have the government give Jenner a state funeral at Westminster Abbey, where he would be interred with other distinguished members of the British Empire. The government debated for nine days, while the remains awaited a decision. Finally, it was decided that Jenner could be buried at Westminster Abbey, but only if his family bore the entire cost of the funeral. An interment in the Abbey implied an expenditure beyond what any private family could afford, and this was particularly true for the Jenner family who were of modest means. Jenner left no large fortune, since he gave freely of his discovery, vaccination, and over the years, his small income from his medical practices in Berkeley and Cheltenham was used to support his family, and to provide for the poor farmers and laborers in the surrounding area of Berkeley.

A burial at Westminster Abbey was not possible. Anyway, Jenner would have wished to be interred in the vault beside his beloved Catharine, in the Berkeley Church, amongst the country people he so loved. And that was, finally, where he was buried, while being prayed over by a small group of his relatives and friends.

For such a great man, his funeral was simple, with his many friends, neighbors and patients from Berkeley and Cheltenham in attendance. Shortly after the ceremony, the doctors of Gloucester began a collection for a statue honoring Jenner. They had hoped that the work would be done by a famous artist, but the funds failed to meet their expectations. Fortunately, a young, relatively unknown, sculptor agreed to produce the statue at a cost that they could afford. The work was finished in September of 1825. It was a fine statue that was erected in the nave of the Gloucester Cathedral among statues of other distinguished gentry of the region.

Doctor Jenner had elated and energized the world with his discovery of how to rid itself of the dreaded and detested smallpox disease. No one would deny that this discovery earned him the honor of a public funeral, with all of its pomp and ceremony, and burial in Westminster Abbey. However, all the local folks knew that Jenner would be much happier to be buried in his beloved Berkeley, in the church that overlooked his home. Before the altar of that chuch, on the floor, is a stone slab covering his burial place. On it is recorded his name and nearby is a stained-glass, decorated window, dedicated to Christ the Healer. Jenner's mission in life also was to heal the sick, but his greatest contribution to humanity was to show those who came after him how to rid the world of one of its greatest evils, smallpox, and thus he earned the right to be known as: The man who saved the world from smallpox.

In the annals of medicine, Jenner holds a unique place. Rarely, if at all, has a medical discovery been accepted so rapidly and completely by so many countries as Jenner's smallpox vaccination. Nor has any doctor so quickly received universal acclamation as Jenner did for his discovery of vaccination. Almost instantaneously, Jenner went from being an unknown country doctor to a highly respected and idolized international medical figure. Once the *Inquiry* was circulated abroad and was translated into numerous languages, vaccination was immediately perceived to be a safe way of preventing smallpox; and it quickly became the standard practice for preventing this horrible disease.

It is not difficult to understand the universal veneration lavished upon Jenner. Smallpox was a worldwide misery which produced suffering, deformity, blindness and death; but most of all, it caused intense fear and trepidation in everyone. No one is certain how long smallpox has been exclusively a human disease; some think at least two thousand years. No matter; it still has killed more people than all the wars combined, since the beginning of recorded time. How many people were badly disfigured or blinded will never be known. Smallpox knew no bounds; it gave no quarter; and compassion, mercy and sympathy were unknown to it. All were equally attacked by it: kings, queens, emperors, royalty, tyrants, warlords, despots; the rich as well as the poor; good people and bad people; believers and non-believers. Smallpox treated all equally and with the same ferocity. It was always there in the background waiting to strike, when people least expected it. If a few words could describe smallpox they are fear, constant fear and apprehension. This is what Jenner's discovery, vaccination, removed from the people of the earth. It is no wonder, then, that he was adored and idolized by all people, most of whom knew nothing more about him than his name.

◆ ◆ ◆

Finally, Jenner's story was finished and the evening was over. Everyone got out of their seats and began walking about the room in order to stretch their leg muscles and get the blood flowing to their frozen feet.

They all were happy, and any small annoyances that occurred during the evening were quickly forgiven. They were satisfied, not because the evening was over, but because they had a sense of accomplishment. They exuded a spirit of cooperation, of brotherhood, which is usually known only to soldiers who cared for each other during a battle.

The men began shaking hands, while the ladies gave each other gentle kisses on the cheeks. Then there was the exchange of comments: "I'm so tired I could sleep for a week," and "I pray that the children will not wake up early today."

EPILOGUE

There is no reason that fictitious characters in a story should not have a life of their own, before and after their life in a book is finished. So, for those who would like know what happened to the imaginary people, I have included something about their lives, because even authors like to know what became of the people that they created.

The Penfields, Lawrence and Iris: It is sad to report that shortly after the story finished, Lawrence, or as he was better known in the story, Prof, died suddenly of a heart attack. Iris grieved for a short time over the Prof's death and then suddenly remarried. Her new spouse is a stuffy old Cambridge don, whose affairs she manages rather handily, much as she did for the Prof. Iris also continues her own active and productive life.

The Foxworths, Cedric and Sarah: Cedric left the Prof's biology department in London and became a dean at a small university in southern England. Cedric was a successful dean, while remaining a rather controversial figure. Sarah accepted a position as an historian at the same university.

The Goldmans, Murray and Ruth: They left England, soon after the story ended, and moved to Canada where he was appointed professor at a leading Canadian university. Shortly after arriving in Canada, Ruth became an active member in the Canadian Jewish community and spent most of her time participating in their charitable and social programs.

The Joneses, James (Jimmy) and Valerie: A year after the story finished, they left London and moved back to Chicago, where Jimmy assumed his position as professor of biology at a Chicago university. Valerie, when she wasn't occupied managing their large family, spent her time reading and doing editorial work. Some years later, Jimmy and Valerie retired and left Chicago for a small, west Texas town, which is on the flight path of migratory birds that he loves to identify and, at times, to count.

Dr. Edward Jenner, the protagonist of this story, rests peacefully in a crypt next to his beloved wife, in a little church in Gloucestershire.

0-595-32957-8

Lightning Source UK Ltd.
Milton Keynes UK
04 April 2011

170343UK00002B/105/A